K

DATE DUE

BRODART.   Cat. No. 23-221

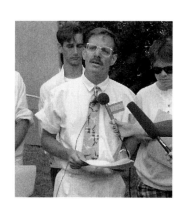

AIDS **ACTIVIST**

Michael Lynch
and the
Politics of Community

ANN SILVERSIDES

Between the Lines
Toronto, Canada

AIDS Activist

First published in Canada in 2003 by
Between the Lines
720 Bathurst Street, Suite #404
Toronto, Ontario M5S 2R4
1-800-718-7201
www.btlbooks.com

National Library of Canada Cataloguing in Publication

Silversides, Ann, 1952–
    AIDS activist : Michael Lynch and the politics of community / Ann Silversides.

Includes bibliographical references and index.
ISBN 1-896357-73-3

    I. AIDS (Disease)— Political aspects. 2. Gay men. I. Title.

RA644.A25S57 2003   362.1'969792   C2003-902225-0

Cover design by David Vereschagin, Quadrat Communications
Front cover photograph by David Vereschagin
Photo of Michael Lynch, opposite title page, courtesy of Philip Hannan
The silhouette image on p.xiii is taken from the "Numbers" poster; see p.135.
Text design by Jennifer Tiberio
Printed in Canada

Between the Lines gratefully acknowledges assistance for its publishing activities from the
Canada Council for the Arts, the Ontario Arts Council, the Government of Ontario through the
Ontario Book Publishers Tax Credit program and through the Ontario Book Initiative, and the
Government of Canada through the Book Publishing Industry Development Program.

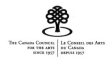
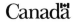

THE CANADA COUNCIL | LE CONSEIL DES ARTS
FOR THE ARTS | DU CANADA
SINCE 1957 | DEPUIS 1957

Canadä

ONTARIO ARTS COUNCIL
CONSEIL DES ARTS DE L'ONTARIO

CONTENTS

FOREWORD

ONE OVERCAST New York afternoon in June 1994, a rented yacht idled under the Brooklyn Bridge. A group of friends, myself included, were gathered on board to carry out a final act of memorial for Michael Lynch. Before Michael died in 1991, he had asked that his ashes be scattered from the bridge that had so inspired one of his favourite poets, Hart Crane. A trademark Michael wish, and so here we were at last, three years later, drawn together in New York for the twenty-fifth anniversary celebrations of the Stonewall riots, the symbolic birth event of the gay liberation movement.

The request had seemed simple enough to carry out (not without some effort and inconvenience, of course) until Michael's son Stefan discovered that the design of the pedestrian walkways made ash-scattering from the bridge virtually impossible. Now what would we do? Finally, someone made the obvious suggestion. Why not use a boat?

Our vessel had taken us to a spot on the East River in the shadow of the Brooklyn Bridge's massive suspension spans. Once moored, we read selections from Michael's favourite poets, lifted glasses of champagne in a toast, and tossed overboard brightly coloured gerberas (one of Michael's favourite flowers). Finally, as the boat picked up speed to return to shore, we took turns dropping Michael's ashes from a container into the river. Then, unexpectedly, lifted by a gust of wind, plumes of fine ash flew back into our faces and clothes, dropping tiny spots on the remaining champagne in our glasses. We contemplated the silly symbolism of this moment, and our tears turned to laughter as we made our way back to dock.

Even during this final act of memorial, it seemed, Michael had once again managed to leave his mark on his friends. I was certainly one of the people who had felt enriched by Michael's friendship over the years. But whose lives beyond his circle of friends did he touch?

An American by birth, Michael moved to Canada in 1971 to take a job teaching English literature at the University of Toronto. In that city he became one of a group of individuals associated with *The*

Body Politic, a gay liberation magazine whose advocacy journalism became an inspiration to activist circles around the world. The decade of the 1970s, punctuated at its end by sensational courtroom trials, chilling police raids, and angry demonstrations, proved to be a valuable training ground for Michael and a cadre of activists schooled in the rough skills of movement journalism and committed to the politics of collective action. The lessons he learned from gay organizing in Toronto during those early years, fuelled by his personal grief over friends suddenly snatched away by AIDS, gave him the vision to inspire others to resist, to organize, and to mourn during the toughest years of the AIDS crisis in Toronto.

Michael did not fit any of the mass media-inspired caricatures of the one-dimensional "activist." His interests were remarkably diverse. In addition to his pioneering pieces of advocacy journalism in *The Body Politic* and his AIDS organizing, Michael taught the first gay studies course at the University of Toronto, founded Gay Fathers of Toronto, edited the first lesbian and gay studies newsletter in North America, launched the first community-based queer studies organization in Canada, and published a book of poetry. He fulfilled a personal fantasy by posing for nude spreads in two gay erotic magazines. He loved to haunt the disco dance floors in New York and Toronto, and threw fabulous parties. Throughout all of this, before he died of AIDS at the age of forty-six, he managed to raise a remarkable son.

In 1982 and 1983, with the arrival of the "mysterious illness," the sudden deaths, and the confusion and fear they brought, Michael Lynch's plea for an organized and calm resistance strategy in the face of the pending crisis helped to shape an entire community's response to AIDS and keep it true to the principles of sexual liberation and democratic organizing. Throughout the worst of the AIDS years in the 1980s, his was one of the primary voices of reason and passion within Toronto's gay community. Michael managed always to bring a calming influence to organizational politics. He understood the different roles that organizations and institutions could strategically play in responding to a health crisis like AIDS. He recognized the need for healing rituals to give public expression to private grief, to commemorate, in his words, "these waves of dying friends." In Michael Lynch's world, there was a place for both mourning and militancy.

Looking back now at those formative years, we can say that the gay community, inspired by the strength and vision of early AIDS activists like Michael Lynch—and there were, of course, countless others who shared in this work—made the right choices in its responses to the epidemic. Its legacy is a network of diverse AIDS service organizations serving the needs of diverse communities. Whole new generations of queer youth have never known anything but the persistent warning theme of AIDS and safer sex running in the background of their lives. Medical advances in drug therapies have prolonged many lives, and AIDS deaths are no longer frequent or inevitable.

Yet in some cases the welcome sense of confidence and entitlement that young people feel today is also creating a less desirable legacy: complacency about condom use and boredom with safer needle and safer sex advice. There is no longer an overwhelming sense of urgency or crisis driving the HIV/AIDS agenda. Rates of infection among young gay men are reportedly on the increase, and the slow attrition of funding for HIV prevention programs barely registers on the media's radar screen.

Are the hard lessons learned in the 1980s portable to the next challenge? Are our various communities ready to rally to meet the next crisis (there is always another crisis)? Is our sense of preparedness dulled? Will we remember—and be inspired by—the example of those early days of AIDS activism? Only time will tell.

In the meantime, the story of a community's response to HIV/AIDS and the role that Michael Lynch and others played in that response is a resilient narrative of hope and inspiration and triumph over adversity. Ann Silversides' account captures personal and political moments from that story, and brings a history already fading from memory back into sharp relief.

ED JACKSON

Ed Jackson has been, at various times over the last thirty years, an editor of The Body Politic, *director of education at the AIDS Committee of Toronto, and a board member of the Toronto Centre for Lesbian and Gay Studies.*

PREFACE

MICHAEL LYNCH said "to write history is to write against death." This book comes out of loss. My cousin Brian Silversides died on April 16, 1996, at age forty-six, from complications related to AIDS. From our teenage years until his death, Brian and I were co-conspirators. We discussed films, theatre, and books, knew each other's friends, confided in each other about love and pain. In the last years of Brian's life, I got to know many of his friends who were HIV-positive or had AIDS.

After Brian died I began writing, as a kind of homage, a column on AIDS issues for *Xtra* in Toronto. I also created a three-hour radio documentary—"Sex, Death and Grief: The Impact of AIDS Losses among Gay Men"—for CBC-Radio's *Ideas* program. (The series aired in May 1997.) The "general public" really had very little idea about the devastation that AIDS had brought to the community of gay men, or about the impact on that community of homophobia and the stigma associated with AIDS. I also came to realize that the story of the early years of the epidemic in Canada had to be documented.

When I interviewed Dr. Philip Berger for the radio documentary, he told the story of a group of friends, "gay hippie types," who were all patients of his. For gay men, their family is very often their friends, and so it was for this group. All of them are now dead except one (who is HIV-negative). Just before one of this circle of friends died, he wondered who would be left to remember them. "You get this sense of almost non-existence," Berger said.

It was Alan Miller at the Canadian Lesbian and Gay Archives in Toronto who set me on the path that I eventually followed. I showed up at the archives, eager with my (overly ambitious) plan to interview AIDS activists across Canada and pull together a nationwide history of early AIDS activism. "You could do worse than to look at Michael Lynch," Miller said. Several months later, I saw the wisdom in this more focused approach. I began reading through the treasure trove of Lynch's diaries, and knew I was on track. I could tell a story that was both personal and political, that revealed the visceral impact of the epidemic and celebrated the activists' spirit of challenge and resistance. Michael Lynch's former wife Gail, and his son, Stefan, were encouraging and helpful to this project. Along the way I had the invaluable help of many of Lynch's friends, whom I interviewed in Toronto, New York, and cyberspace. All were positive and forthcoming, but among them I would like to single out Rick Bébout, Alan Miller, and Michael Hulton, who were good-natured as I kept bothering them with questions. I also thank the volunteers at the CLGA, where I spent many evenings rummaging through papers.

After the initial solitary stages of research and writing, a book becomes a community affair and so I thank my husband, Phil Hall, for his support (from the very beginning) and insightful commentary on early drafts; my editor, Robert Clarke, for a broad vision and a meticulous attention to detail from which I and the book benefited; BTL staff members Paul Eprile, Jennifer Tiberio, and Peter Steven; and designer David Vereschagin for his inspired cover design. I also acknowledge the support of the Canada Council, Ontario Arts Council (Writers' Reserve Program), and Toronto Arts Council.

Two of Brian's HIV-positive friends, artist Rycke Pothier and AIDS activist Peter Wood, became my good friends. On July 9, 2001—the ten-year anniversary of Michael Lynch's death—his son Stefan, who now lives in San Francisco, hosted a Toronto reunion of his father's care team. After that gathering, which I attended as a special guest (I had not been on the care team), I bicycled home to news that Rycke Pothier had died that afternoon. Three months later, Peter Wood died. "All the boys," as Peter used to say, "all the boys who've died."

This book is for all of them.

ANN SILVERSIDES

NOTE ON THE TEXT: In most cases quotations from Michael Lynch's diaries are set in *Scala Sans Italic*. The main text is set in Scala.

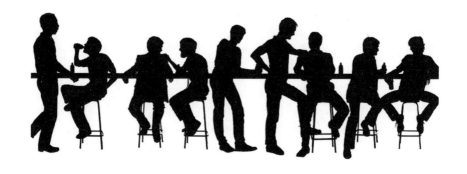

one

A POLITICAL BODY

"JULY 3 MARKS THE DAY most people remember as the beginning of the thing," Michael Lynch wrote in 1982. *"The muggy first day of a crazy holiday weekend on Manhattan and at Fire Island."*[1]

Michael Lynch knew it was muggy on Fire Island that July holiday weekend in 1981 because he was there. Since 1978 he had been spending summers at the island, taking time away from his home in Toronto, where he had been living and teaching at the University of Toronto for almost a decade. The gay resort of Fire Island was less than two hours by train and ferry or water taxi from downtown New York City. It got its name, apparently, from the warning fires built there by nineteenth-century whalers, and it was home to two enclaves— Cherry Grove ("the Grove") and the more affluent Pines. Lynch rented houses in The Pines with a shifting group of friends and acquaintances, and in 1981 he felt lucky to be able to spend more than three months there, from late May to early September. The extensive free time was one of the perks of being a English professor.

Gay life at The Pines had its rituals. The beach, of course, was the highlight during the day. Then, about six in the evening, the Tea-Dance began at a restaurant attached to the hotel. It lasted until about 8 p.m., when most island residents wandered off for dinner. Midnight was the time to head to the Ice Palace dance hall for the disco, which continued into the early morning. Drugs—especially

1

uppers and poppers to better appreciate the disco—were in ready supply, and sexual exploits peppered the landscape.

Lynch embraced this life, although that particular summer he kept his sexual exploits to a minimum because he was writing a novel and cultivating a long-distance romance with a man back in Toronto. For much of his adult life, Lynch kept a series of small black notebook-diaries, numbered sequentially, in which he recorded the events of everyday life. By 1981 he was into diary number 20, and on his way home to Toronto in early September that year, he noted that he was already missing The Pines' predominantly gay surroundings, its gay texture. *"Again I'm leaving to be around straights, be in an invisible minority."* In Toronto, he thought, you had to *"look hard to discern other gays."* On Fire Island gays were a given, which was "splendid." Still, he thought, there was a noticeable limitation on who could or couldn't come to the place. Who couldn't come? Well, Fire Island was for the well-heeled, the "gay haute bourgeoisie," as Lynch's New York friend Herb Spiers put it.

Late in the summer, on August 31, Lynch brought his nine-year-old son to the island and for the last week of his stay on Fire Island he tried unsuccessfully to mix parenting and partying. *"Stefan had another day of misery,"* he wrote in his diary. *"The party especially was a bad time for him."* Stefan kept saying things like *"I didn't have a good time,"* *"People keep bumping into me,"* *"No one noticed me,"* and *"People stared at me like I was funny—what's a kid doing here?"* Lynch summed it up: *"His week has been very bad."* Later on, Lynch's friend Herb Spiers would note that in the late 1970s/early 1980s many gay activists "were leery of children, because, well, what were they but the embodiment of the nuclear family, which at the time was the central place of attack in gay liberationist theory of the causes of gay oppression."[2] Lynch was something of a pioneer in opposing that trend.

Somewhat oddly though, despite all of its interesting details, Lynch's diary that summer made no mention of the mysterious new illness that was causing a ripple of concern in the community—the one he would be writing about (*"July 3 marks the day . . ."*) more than a year later. Indeed, many accounts of the AIDS epidemic in North America would begin by taking note of an article that appeared in *The New York Times* on that day—July 3, 1981—under the headline

"Rare Cancer Seen in 41 Homosexuals." The article, based on a report from the Centers for Disease Control in Atlanta, referred to cases of Kaposi's sarcoma (KS), a disfiguring cancer involving the lymph nodes or skin. Typically found only in men of age fifty and over, the cancer had suddenly appeared in healthy young men; the mean age in the new outbreak was thirty-nine years of age. An even earlier CDC report, on June 5, had also generated coverage in the mainstream media (*Los Angeles Times* and *San Francisco Chronicle*) as well as in the *New York Native*, a publication serving the gay community of New York. That June CDC item described five severe pneumonia cases involving young homosexual men; their sexual orientation was the only thing they had in common. The cases were notable because the illness, pneumocystis carinii pneumonia (PCP), usually occurred only in newborns or people who had undergone organ transplants and were taking immunosuppressive drugs.[3]

But for most gay men in New York, it was the article in the *Times* that first got their attention. And at the very end of that summer, on Labour Day weekend, playwright Larry Kramer and friends began sounding the alarm on Fire Island. The men, who would form the core of a group called Gay Men's Health Crisis in New York, leafleted the island with brochures that included the first *New York Native* feature article, "Cancer in the Gay Community," from July. The *Native* reported that of forty-one men stricken with KS in New York and California over the past two years, eight were now dead. Kramer himself wrote an article, published in the *Native* in late August, which opened: "It's difficult to write this without sounding alarmist or too emotional or just plain scared."[4]

Lynch, still on the island on Labour Day weekend, recorded nothing in his diary about these now famous events. Even though he mentioned reading the *New York Native*, Lynch made no reference to the "new gay cancer," as it was already being called. But an earlier diary entry, for May 31 of that same year, does contain one ominous passage: *"Tea was not too crowded, with several friendly faces. Victor spoke—1st time I've seen him since last summer: looking very pale, thin. Two friends, one very close, recently died and much disturbance for him."*

Dunn, Dot, Dad, and Base

Accompanied by his wife Gail, American-born Michael Lynch had arrived in Toronto in 1971. At age twenty-seven, Lynch was moving north to take up a position teaching English at St. Michael's College in the University of Toronto. He and Gail had met at the University of Iowa in 1968, when they were both students. She was completing a Masters degree in English literature, and he was working on a Ph.D., writing his thesis on poet Wallace Stevens. He had a prestigious NDEA (National Defense Education Act) fellowship, which paid all his living expenses. When Gail first met him, Lynch was a redhead with freckles. "He had long unkempt hair, his shoes were pointy toed, bought at Goodwill," she said later. For Gail Jones, who had grown up in an upper-middle-class Chicago suburb, the figure of this aspiring poet of the sixties held a curious attraction. "He ran around in wrinkled jeans, wearing an army jacket and baggy sweaters," she said. "He lived in a farm house, growing his own food."[5]

The two got married in Iowa City on July 5, 1969. In keeping with the times, the wedding ceremony was suitably unconventional, with readings from Martin Buber, Eldridge Cleaver, and Antoine de Saint-Exupéry as well as poets William Carlos Williams and James Tate. The music was Otis Redding, the Beatles, and Arcangelo Corelli. Fellow students from the university's famed creative writing school composed poems especially for the occasion. The couple arranged for the ceremony to be written up for the *Dunn Courier*, the newspaper from Lynch's North Carolina hometown, in a style appropriate to that publication:

> The bride wore an informal mini-gown of bridal cotton lace over taffeta fashioned with an Empire waist and an A-line skirt. The bodice was adorned with lace-covered buttons which climaxed in a Puritan collar. . . . The groom wore bell-bottom trousers of white linen and a midnight blue shirt with Edwardian ruffles and collar.

The marriage in itself was also unconventional. Lynch had been attracted to men, and aware of this attraction, for years. As a teenager, while still at home in Dunn, he had spoken to his church minister about his feelings, trying to sort things out. At the University of Iowa his feelings for the opposite sex remained strong, if not acted upon. While there he was enrolled in a government-sponsored counselling program that aimed, literally, at "straightening out" homosexuals—changing their orientation from homosexual to heterosexual. The program, not surprisingly, met with no success—though it did help him avoid the U.S. draft. But by that time, too, he had become influenced by his Oberlin College mentor, Professor Thomas Whitaker, an academic with a wife and four children, and he aspired to be the sort of academic "model family man" that he saw in Whitaker. When he met Gail he found a kind of soul-mate. Gail also wanted a family, and she didn't find Lynch's declared attraction to men threatening. At university she had sexual relations with both men and women and had few expectations of a Good Housekeeping-style of married life. "Michael talked about being interested in men *and* wanting to be married. We just understood each other," she said years later.

Lynch had grown up in Dunn, a town of about 8,000 with a clear division in its makeup: half the population was white, and the other half Black. He and his younger brother Pat had been adopted by Dot (born Dorothy Driver) and Pat Lynch—though the boys were not related by birth. Their father, a mechanical engineer, owned Lynch Manufacturing Co., a machine shop. But Pat Lynch had his problems. He struggled with alcoholism, and for the last several years of his life he was in and out of treatment centres. Later on Michael would tell his own son about those days, about what it was like to take friends home after school and find his father *"in a bed of puke, blinds closed mid-afternoon. How I would be torn apart by even slight tension in the family, and it was seldom slight."* During that time Lynch's mother discouraged him from expressing his feelings to her, and frequently told him he was "too sensitive." He took refuge in playing the piano. *"All my feelings were monstrously strong, powerful, far beyond anyone else's ability to deal w/them, and so I could only 'express' them in piano music,"* he later wrote of that time.

Lynch's father died, at age fifty-seven, on March 22, 1960, at the Rex Hospital in Raleigh, N.C., from the effects of the addiction. Michael Lynch was fifteen years old. He was instructed not to mention his father's name in the family home. Later Stefan would speculate that this experience, the attempted obliteration of memory, was part of what inspired his father to keep journals and save all his correspondence—to generate and save evidence of his life.

His mother's mother, whom he called "Mammy," lived in town, and both generations of Driver women were strong and resourceful. Dot, Michael would say, "hated weakness." She took over the failing family business and turned it into a thriving enterprise after her husband's death. His mother, Lynch later told his diary, *"let me make the key decisions of my life and even when it was difficult supported them, and more than once took scorn for them and yet loved me without regard."* She maddened Michael "with her silliness" and awed him "with her stature." She taught him to treasure friends and dancing.

Michael kept busy with school and the other things that kids do. At age seven, when he showed an interest in music, his mother had promptly bought him a 1906 Steinway piano. He began taking lessons and continued to study piano throughout university. (Later, one of the great disappointments in his life was when he failed to be admitted to the Oberlin Music Academy.) As a young boy Lynch spent a good deal of time with Mabel, his father's sister (whom Lynch called Base), and her live-in companion, Esther. Both women were schoolteachers, and among other things they taught young Michael how to cook and to garden—two domestic pursuits of no interest to his mother—and he became a superb cook and a devoted gardener. When Base died in 1961 the loss was the second devastating blow in slightly more than a year. Years later, in 1979, he wrote that as a child he believed Base and Esther were his real parents; and in 1980 he wrote that the great fact of his life, bearing on everything, was *"the death of Base in 1961, forever leaving, abandoning me."*

Michael was a youth leader in the Hood Memorial Christian Church and a page at the North Carolina legislature in Raleigh. He spent two summers teaching poor Black children to read and write. "His mother always stressed the importance of being a good citizen," Gail recalled. "She was outgoing, assertive, and without prejudice. You could also see those qualities in Michael." After high school Lynch went off to university in other small towns—first Oberlin College in Oberlin (population 8,600), and then he followed his mentor, Professor Whitaker, to Goddard College in Plainfield,

Vermont (population 1,000). At university Lynch identified more with the counterculture of the 1960s than with leftist student politics, but the political concerns of "good citizenry" would soon return.

Hidden from Lynch was information about his birth parents. Much later, in Toronto on his thirty-ninth birthday, a year after his mother died, he wrote about his birth mother:

> *And, biking across College today and down Ross St (which always makes me happy) with the lowering sun casting gabled shadows from the west side houses in squares and triangles all the way down the street, I thought of that woman who on a Sunday in August 1944 gave birth to a boy and gave him away: is she still alive? Does she think of that boy today? Does she think that I may think of her when I look in the mirror and say, "are these her brows? Her cheekbones and chin line? Did she sculpt this head, impel these fingers to the piano keys where they, blood rushed, are happiest?" Two mothers, twice blest, twice separated, twice lonely, twice a part and apart.*

Lynch's former student and friend George Poland said that it was only after Dot died that Michael thought seriously about trying to find his birth mother. But in the end Lynch decided that even though his adoptive mother was dead, it would dishonour her memory in his hometown of Dunn if he were to seek out his biological mother. And so he never did initiate a search for his biological parents. Like other adoptees, though, Lynch did have his fantasies. He told his diary that perhaps his real father was the poet Wallace Stevens, who impregnated a young woman on a trip to North Carolina.

Part of that decision not to search revolved around his strong roots in the relations and town of his childhood. Still, after he left Dunn he shed his Southern accent and remade himself from a "Mike" into a "Michael." According to Stefan, Lynch also wanted very much to be a Yankee. "He had an absolutely standard accent. He was one of those people who could return to the south and not change [his accent] at all," Stefan recalled. "My dad would never once say y'all, it was such a point of pride."

But in his dreams (recorded in his diaries) he returned again and again to that emotional and physical landscape, going over his relationships with his mother, his grandmother, and Base. Later on, in regular sessions with bioenergetic therapist Sage Walker, Lynch also devoted much time to exploring his connections—and lack of them—with his father.

Gay liberation in the "human rights decade"

In Toronto Michael and Gail settled into an apartment on the seventeenth floor of a building on Walmer Road near Bloor Street, near the University of Toronto in the area called "The Annex." After a life so far spent in small towns, he was thrilled to be living in the heart of a large city. Their son Stefan was born on January 9, 1972. Lynch was a delighted father, particularly so because, as an adoptee, he now had his first known blood relative. Just after Stefan was born, Lynch was walking up Avenue Road and met a friend. Lynch took the occasion to tell the friend the good news by bursting into song: "For unto us a child is born."[6]

When Stefan was nine months old, the Lynches set up housekeeping in a solid Tudor-style two-storey house on Roehampton Avenue in North Toronto, a middle-class enclave. But the shape of the marriage quickly changed. Lynch belatedly came to realize that his real desire was to lead the life of a gay man. He had his first sexual encounter with a man when Stefan was nine months old. Gail had been "on the grand tour," showing Stefan off to relatives in the United States. "When I got off the plane, Michael was glowing," she remembered. Lynch told her he had just slept with a man for the first time. "I was so happy for him," Gail said. "Neither one of us thought of it as threatening our marriage at that point."

Stefan was a toddler when Lynch began attending meetings of GATE, the Gay Alliance Toward Equality, and still Gail did not feel that the marriage was under threat. "He was so intent on us being a family," she said. With the birth of his son Lynch may well have been accomplishing something important to him—fatherhood—that would have been much more difficult as a strictly gay man; that done, he could now explore his attraction to men. But the marriage continued more uneasily after Stefan's birth, and eventually, five years later, Gail moved out of their home at 435 Roehampton, and Michael's male lover at the time, Bill Lewis, moved in. Lewis, a microbiologist, was also teaching at the University of Toronto—he had taken up a teaching post there in 1977, at the age of twenty-seven.

Around that time Lynch's mother was visiting Toronto, and he told her about his homosexuality. Gail Lynch was there and heard the conversation. The first thing Michael's mother said was, "Well, I still love you." As Gail said later, "We're not talking about a young woman here, she was in her sixties." The second thing Michael's mother said was, "I don't know much about this, you're going to have to tell me."

Meanwhile, in those first years in Toronto, Lynch became deeply immersed in gay politics and issues as well as in a gay lifestyle. In 1973 he began writing for *The Body Politic*, a newsmagazine run as a non-profit collective. *The Body Politic* had an international reputation. Its paid circulation was never more than about 9,000, but it was highly regarded and influential among English-speaking gay activist circles around the world—and a magnet and training ground for gay liberation activists. Members of the collective—the paper never had more than two paid staff—would go on to become key leaders in the early days of AIDS. It was, collective member Rick Bébout recalled years later, not just a newsmagazine but "a kind of political party, a movement, and a kind of aesthetic voice . . . an activist academy."[7]

At the same time in those early years, Lynch was very much part of the St. Michael's College community. He and Gail went to church every Sunday at the college, attending an alternative mass held in a basement and featuring guitars and gospel-singing. In the 1973–74 academic year Lynch organized a poetry series at the college, bringing John Ashbery and Yevgeny Yevtushenko, among others, to the campus. Paul McGrath, who was cultural affairs commissioner at the student union and helped with the series, was a student of Lynch's. "Poetry was a passion with him, a joy. Nobody before had shown me the secrets, the mission of poetry; he opened it up in three weeks."

In 1974 Lynch created a course on gay studies to be offered at night through the University of Toronto's continuing education department. "New Perspectives on the Gay Experience" was the first such course at a Canadian university, and featured guest lecturers theologian Gregory Baum, professor and biographer Phyllis Gross-kurth, psychiatrist David Berger, and sociologist John Alan Lee. But the publicity around the course as well as Lynch's public profile as a rising gay activist did not sit well with authorities at St. Michael's—after all, it was a Roman Catholic college. A showdown with the college principal proved traumatic; Lynch had dreams about the event for years afterwards. He was told that he could stay at the downtown college only if he became silent on gay issues. After long and difficult negotiations, he was eventually offered the alternative of tenure and a transfer to Erindale College, a suburban U of T campus. He accepted.

Lynch would call the 1970s the "Human Rights Decade" because of the push for legal rights for gays and lesbians that was gaining momentum. It was only in 1969 in Canada that Criminal Code amendments had decriminalized sexual acts ("buggery" and "gross indecency") between consenting adults over age twenty-one and in private. The legislation was not, however, universally viewed as a great victory, because the age of consent for homosexual sexual acts was older than it was for heterosexual sexual acts—a fact that prompted the North American Conference of Homophile Organizations to send a formal protest to Prime Minister Pierre Trudeau.[8] South of the border, most observers credit the 1969 Stonewall riots with giving birth to the gay liberation movement and a period of heightened gay activism. In late June that year, New York police raided the Stonewall Inn, a gay bar, and, for the first time, patrons and others fought back. Young members of the Mattachine Society, a homosexual rights organization, subsequently organized and created the Gay Liberation Front, which had links with the Black Panthers and Students for a Democratic Society (sDs).[9] All of this activity was influenced by the surging radical politics of the 1960s: the civil rights, ban-the bomb, and anti-war movements, and women's liberation (as it was then called). As writer Vanessa Baird points out, "As feminists examined and challenged sexism, and black activists fought racism under slogans such as 'Black is Beautiful,' it was indeed time to challenge the prejudice against homosexuals."[10]

The gay liberation movement spread north. Four months after Stonewall, the University of Toronto Homophile Association was formed, and on August 28, 1971, the first large-scale public gay demonstration was held in Canada. The protest, for gay and lesbian rights, was staged at Parliament Hill in Ottawa by Toronto Gay Action, a gay liberation group that grew out of the Community Homophile Association of Toronto, which in turn had grown out of the U of T group. (When Toronto Gay Action disbanded in 1973, its activist role was taken over by GATE.)[11]

But with the emerging gay rights movement came a backlash against gay rights from the religious right. In the United States the charge was led by Anita Bryant, an entertainer known for appearing in television advertisements promoting Florida Orange Juice, and Rev. Jerry Falwell. Their Canadian allies included Rev. Ken Campbell, of Renaissance Canada, who invited Bryant to bring her "Save the Children" campaign to Canada. Her 1977 visit to Ontario prompted the largest gay and lesbian demonstration to that date, with eight hundred people marching up Yonge Street in Toronto.[12]

In that decade Lynch established himself as a gay leader in Toronto. He was a founding member of the Toronto Gay Academic Union in 1975 and a founding member in 1978 of Gay Fathers Toronto. That same year, he was chair of the Committee to Defend John Damien (a jockey fired for his sexual orientation), and he was active with GATE, which, for example, lobbied the Ontario Human Rights Commission for the inclusion of sexual orientation in the province's Human Rights Code. When he was ready to spearhead a new organization, he would often begin by writing a feature article on the issue in *The Body Politic*. His article "Defending Damien," for instance, appeared in October 1977, and "Forgotten Fathers: Gay Men with Children May Be More Common—and More Important to All of Us—Than Anyone Has Yet Guessed" appeared in the magazine in April 1978.[13]

"Forgotten Fathers" appeared well before Lynch's experience (in September 1981) with his son Stefan on Fire Island—an experience that had probably occurred at least a few times before. When Lynch wrote the article, the attitude among gay men and lesbians towards parents was very different than it would be two decades or so later. Sheri Zernentsch, a friend of Stefan's, argued in a 1998 thesis that anti-gay lobbies in the 1970s widened the gap between gay and heterosexual lifestyle: "Many gay men responded by veering away from interaction with children. Gay culture soon became a culture that rejected children and other dependants, as activists in the gay and lesbian rights movement advocated for gay social freedom through a culture of sexual liberation and increased individualism." Like Stefan, Zernentsch had a gay father, and when she and her brother went out in public with him they often came up against the verbal rejections of anything related to or involving children, including the "what are you doing here?" attitude. "Terms such as 'breeders' became commonplace ways to slander heterosexuals and heterosexual culture," she wrote. To her, Michael Lynch's pioneering work was "certainly the exception."[14] Stefan, who as a young adult founded an organization called Children of Lesbians and Gays Everywhere, said he was very lucky: "My dad figured out how to both be a dad and a gay man. In my generation, that is extremely rare."

By the end of the decade Lynch was arguing in the pages of *The Body Politic* that the political battles of the 1970s to obtain human rights protection had brought gay life to public consciousness in a way hitherto unknown. "Homosexuality is now a public issue, politicized even in the non-gay press, no longer clamped into the sin/sickness/deviance syndrome." But the fight, he thought, also had another aspect. It had created a gay community "that sees itself, and is seen by others, as a political 'minority.'" And the very success of the movement in achieving human rights protections might well prove detrimental to gay activism. It could lull the community into a kind of lethargy, and lead it to abandon its radical ambitions for fundamental changes in society.[15]

In the late 1970s and early 1980s the gay community and its flagship newsmagazine in Toronto found themselves mobilizing against outside threats. One of those came in 1977, with the brutal murder in July of Emanuel Jaques, a twelve-year-old shoeshine boy in downtown Toronto. The murder was widely referred to in the press as a homosexual killing, and a kind of fear and loathing descended on the city. According to Ed Jackson, a founding member of the *Body Politic* collective, the event was particularly frightening because it was difficult if not impossible to make the sharp distinction that the murder had been carried out by a group with little connection to the local gay community. Just three weeks before the murder, a report had recommended that sexual orientation be included in the Ontario Human Rights Code. That recommendation quickly "went out the window" in the wake of the Jaques killing. The attitude seemed to be, "If we give them more freedoms and rights, this is the kind of thing that will result," Jackson told a federal inquiry.[16]

Four months later, *The Body Politic* published an article on sex between boys and men. Police raided the magazine's offices, seized its subscription list, and laid charges against Pink Triangle Press, which owned the magazine, and the author of the article, Gerald Hannon. There followed a concerted effort "to discredit the news-magazine as a sort of sleazy underground rag," Jackson said. Toronto mayor John Sewell spoke at a rally in support of the magazine and freedom of speech. The publication lost its government grants and faced two full trials. It was acquitted twice on charges of distributing "immoral, indecent and scurrilous" material. But the trials, which dragged on from 1978 to 1983, had "detrimental effects, I think, on our ability to respond to other things sometimes," Jackson remarked.[17]

More was to follow. On December 9, 1978, Toronto police raided the Barracks bathhouse and seized membership lists, despite the 1969 changes in the law that decriminalized sexual acts between consenting adults in private. Bathhouses, it was argued, were not private places, but rather could be classified as bawdy houses, and the police acted under those Criminal Code provisions. Police telephoned school boards to inform them about teachers who were arrested in the bath raids—an initiative that underscored an apparent belief on the part of the police "that homosexuals are all pedophiles at heart," commented George Hislop, a gay community leader. In 1979 the police raided another bathhouse, the Hot Tub Club. In the 1980 city election campaign Mayor Sewell endorsed Hislop's candidacy for alderman of Ward 6, and homosexuality became an election issue. Both men were defeated in the Nov. 10 election.[18]

Perhaps the most dramatic turn of affairs came on Feb. 5, 1981, when the city police co-ordinated a huge raid on the bathhouses. They charged 289 men as "found-ins" and took crowbars and sledge-hammers to the bathhouse premises. The next night, in the first of several such protests, three thousand people took to the streets in downtown Toronto as gay leaders organized a huge demonstration.

The event became known as Toronto's Stonewall. Lynch wrote at 3:20 a.m. on February 7: "*Back an hour ago fr/the anti-cop demo, where I was pounded once in the head by a thug cop on the steps of Queen's Park . . . so many cops . . . all laughing and secure in the knowledge that full state power is behind them . . . Locked doors at home.*"

Prominent Torontonians such as Sewell, author Margaret Atwood, and journalist Laurier LaPierre, as well as organizations such as the Toronto District School Board, the Canadian Civil Liberties Union, the Metro Labour Council, and the Intercity Church Council, also protested the heavy-handed police action.[19]

It was in the wake of this charged political atmosphere that AIDS began to emerge as an issue in Toronto, and the preceding events had two important consequences. Firstly, having just survived a major attack by the authorities, the gay community had a heightened resistance to any attempts to attack or disparage gay men. By that time, too, the members of *The Body Politic* collective had learned to be highly sceptical about media coverage of events and issues affecting gay men. "We had a kind of fixation with the media at the time," Ed Jackson pointed out. "We did not trust them."

Secondly, the community had built new organizations. Out of the Dec. 9, 1978, police raids on the Barracks bathhouse came a new organization, the Right to Privacy Committee (originally called the December 9 Defence Fund).[20] The work that had been done to respond to the raids, including the Right to Privacy Committee's co-ordinated effort, meant that when it came time to organize around AIDS, the gay community had a good working model for political response.

Toronto: gays in health care

In fall 1981, when Michael and Stefan returned from Fire Island to 435 Roehampton Avenue in North Toronto to begin a new academic and school year, the spectre of a new, scary illness was largely absent. But many U.S. gay publications, like the *New York Native, The Advocate,* and *Gay Community News,* carried regular articles about the new illness throughout the rest of 1981 and well into 1982. They were all readily available in Toronto at the gay bookstore Glad Day, then housed on Yonge Street just north of Wellesley, near the city's emerging "gay ghetto."

The first article in *The Body Politic* about the "mysterious new illness" appeared in the September 1981 issue: "'Gay' Cancer and Burning Flesh: The Media Didn't Investigate." It began: "Three recent news reports carried by major newspaper and news media throughout North America have demonstrated a persistent capacity for major distortions in their coverage of gay-related issues." The article compared reports of the "gay cancer" with contemporaneous, sensational mainstream media reports on homosexual sadomasochism. It catalogued "errors of fact" in the initial *New York Times* article. For example, while the *Times* said the cases of Kaposi's sarcoma were "rapidly fatal and largely incurable," *The Body Politic* article asserted that KS is "one of the forms of cancer easiest to cure." It continued: "The most pernicious section of the article, however, is the manner in which it suggests a causal link between the sex lives of gay men and KS."[21] Ever suspicious of the mass media, the *Body Politic* collective members were alert to anything that smacked of homophobia.

Robert Wallace recalled that he and his contemporaries, who had lived through the 1970s and in particular the bathhouse raids, were "sceptical of issues that seemed dubiously linked to gay men. A gay-specific virus? We thought, 'Oh, come on.' It's easy to discriminate against us and easy to spread panic among gay men. The way we saw it, science and medicine were trying to figure out a way to stop us from our sexual hijinks. The climate here was, they're out to stop us, to close the baths. Now they're going to use this disease as an excuse—to panic gay men to self-regulate and to close down the conduit for self-discovery and community-building. There was a reluctance to buy into the scaremongering."

Within a month, at least within the pages of *The Body Politic*, the response from gay activists had become more measured. Bill Lewis and Dr. Randall (Randy) Coates, who was working at the Hassle Free Clinic in Toronto, co-wrote the second *Body Politic* article on the new illness: "Moral Lessons; Fatal Cancer," a full-page feature that appeared in the October 1981 issue. "For most of us, deciding to have sex with other men has meant choosing to risk social disapproval, legal harassment, clap, crabs and syphilis," the article began. "But not cancer, and not death. At least, not until now." The article acknowledged that KS appeared to be much more aggressive in gay men. It also outlined the current hypotheses used to explain the decrease in immune function characteristic of those who suffered from the dangerous opportunistic infections KS and pneumocystis carinii pneumonia. Was immune damage the result of organisms like cytomegalovirus, which "seems to be sexually transmitted," drugs used to treat sexually transmitted diseases, or the use of recreational drugs?

Interestingly, the Lewis and Coates feature ended by arguing that undue attention was being paid to the new illness because it involved homosexuals. "We must endure the publicity which sensationalises another 'gay disease' knowing that if the 26 men with KS had been kidney transplant recipients instead of gay men, no articles would have appeared in the New York Times or The Globe and Mail . . ."

It wouldn't be long, though, before the rallying cry became the *lack* of attention—and research money—devoted by authorities to the illness *precisely because* it involved primarily gay men. Both Lewis and Coates went on to play key roles in the fight against AIDS. Coates himself was a member of Gays in Health Care, a Toronto organization that by the fall of 1981 had begun to track the issue locally. Stephen Atkinson, at the time a psychiatrist in training, had formed the group when he moved to Toronto from Montreal in the summer of 1980. Initially comprising a handful of medical doctors, Gays in Health Care soon opened up to all gay health professionals. Topics for early discussions included sexually transmitted diseases, including hepatitis B, which was then the "new kid on the block," as well as addictions, coming out, and gay mental health, Atkinson said. In June 1981 Atkinson and colleague Richard Isaac had gone to the annual meeting of the Bay Area Physicians for Human Rights (BAPHR), an organization primarily of gay and lesbian doctors. "This was the first time I had ever heard of Kaposi's," Atkinson recalled later of that trip to San Francisco. "I remember feeling an odd alarm in myself and around me as these cases were presented to us."

At the conference Atkinson happened to sit next to a well-known San Francisco public health MD, Selma Dritz, and when presenters on the stage were talking about case reports, Dritz would whisper updates on those cases to the person beside her. "I remember clearly as she included Montreal as one of the cities reporting a case," Atkinson said. At the time the Montreal case—which involved a young gay man from Montreal who was diagnosed in New York—had not been officially reported.[22]

By that time there were reports of 213 cases of the illnesses in the United States: "86 with Kaposi's, 91 with pneumocystis carinii pneumonia, 18 with both and 18 with other opportunistic infections such as disseminated mycobacteria and herpes simplex, central nervous system toxoplasmosis and cryptococcal meningitis," which were considered to be part of the same problem.[23] The first Canadian case of the new condition would be reported in the March 27, 1982, issue of *Canada Diseases Weekly Report*. A gay man in Windsor had entered hospital on January 5, and died Feb. 18. He had suffered from PCP.[24]

In its March/April 1982 newsletter Gays in Health Care included an illustrated article on Kaposi's sarcoma.[25] Its May/June issue provided abstracts of medical press reports on KS and Gay-Related Immunodeficiency Syndrome. In July 1982 the mysterious new syndrome was dubbed the Acquired Immune Deficiency Syndrome, or AIDS. By the time its September/October issue appeared, the Gays in Health Care newsletter was telling its readers, "We are sure you have all been hearing about if not reading the publicity on AIDS in the gay and non-gay media recently." By then the syndrome was being found in more and more non-gay people, such as a number of Haitians and three hemophiliacs. "The clues are still scant but point further in the direction of an infectious cause, perhaps a blood-borne agent." Evidence was also indicating that a forewarning symptom of AIDS could be "generalized lymphadenopathy in otherwise healthy persons." As a result, Toronto's Hassle Free Clinic had arranged a protocol to follow such cases, which included, if appropriate, performing lymphocyte function studies. The Clinic specialized in sexual health and counted many gay men among its clientele.

"A sense of strong but complex moral response . . ."

Until the summer of 1982, Lynch did not record, in his diaries, any of his thinking about the "gay cancer." He would most likely have come into contact with news of the disease much earlier—especially because over the Christmas holidays of 1981 he had been in New York City and gone to Larry Kramer's home for some Chinese food. The outspoken playwright was "nicer" than he had thought he would be, Lynch told his diary. By that point Kramer had raised the alarm and was very much involved in the issue through the Gay Men's Health Crisis, which he had helped to found early that fall.

In New York on the evening of July 9, 1982, Lynch visited Larry Okin, a friend from Fire Island who was in hospital. Okin had undergone a spinal tap and a number of other painful tests to find out what was happening with him. During that weekend visit to New York and The Pines, Lynch reported *"fewer people on the Island,"* but attributed that fact to the recession. On the ninth of August he reported, *"Larry is weak, lesioned and pessimistic."* The lesions are a clear reference to Kaposi's sarcoma. But there was speculation that Larry might also have tuberculosis. Around the same time Lynch also discovered that another friend, Blair Swain, might also have KS.

It was probably during the July visit that Lynch interviewed Larry Okin, Bruce Schentes (Larry's partner), and their friend Michael Cohen for "Living with Kaposi's," his first major feature article on AIDS in *The Body Politic*. *"I must get at the Larry Okin piece,"* he wrote on August 25. Lynch was trying to work out how he would write the piece.

> In the article, a sense of strong but complex moral response, responsibility—Towards the Larrys and Blairs and towards all the rest of us who are really scared by the real things and by unreal, or unknown, things. And morally objecting to those who would amplify the scare needlessly and heedlessly, use the scare as a vehicle for anti-sex. . . . What is special here is that we form a community which is being associated, in our own and in the public minds, with cancer.

The problem was that even before the health crisis gays were already being seen, and treated, as "a cancer on society, illness as metaphor"—pointing to a phrase made famous by writer Susan Sontag—which meant that the health problems would have a special effect on the whole community. The "gay lifestyle" itself had come under attack in article after article in *The Advocate*. Some of the community's best writers and leaders were already engaged in political, fundraising, and public relations activities that were no doubt humanitarian, Lynch thought, but that work was still accepting "without challenge the notion that somehow gayness itself is cancerous." The whole business of the "gay plague," he believed, had become "the most vicious anti-gay campaign, in its effects, since Anita Bryant's."

On the last day of August Michael Lynch's brother Pat telephoned urging him to come to Dunn as soon as he could. Dot, who had been unwell for several months, had slipped into a coma and was in intensive care. On the morning of that same day, Lynch had received a letter from Dot. She lamented her handwriting with a marginal note, "forgive," and sent a clipping of a UPI story on AIDS in homosexuals. *"Life works its way into my writing so neatly I don't believe there are, any more, 'coincidences,'"* he noted.[26]

He made the trip to Dunn, and at his mother's bedside wrote a great deal in his diary about what was happening to his mother and himself, and sketching outlines for the article on AIDS. The first-hand experience of his mother's dying clearly influenced his perspective and thinking on AIDS. *"Will this experience, as it demystifies dying for me, also deglamorize it?"* He hoped that his mother would experience *"a sweet slipping into nothingness,"* but what he got instead was *"a cruel senseless sequence of insults to her, and her body."*

"Mama," as he called her, died a few weeks later, on September 26. *"Today feels like the first day of my adulthood,"* he told his diary. Lynch had returned to Toronto on September 8—Stefan was starting school—and went back to Dunn on the 27th. Later he wrote:

> *How little I felt, riding by the grave tonight after dark (illegally) and stealing a yellow rose and some foliage from the casket spray, that she was there. And how little the talk of the soul and the resurrection of the body convinces me, interests me. I'm so conscious of—saturated with—human experience that the here and now, or rather*

the here and us, most—indeed only—fits for me. I have none of the mysticism I felt after Base's and Daddy's deaths, removed as I then was, from the dying. Now, with the dying, I feel the merely human is enough, More than enough.

Passing through New York on the way back from his mother's funeral, Lynch visited Okin and met another KS patient, who had no medical insurance. So far his treatment had cost $60,000, which his parents had paid for. *"Larry had been lucky,"* Lynch noted. *"His employer had covered his more than $100,000 in medical bills for him."*

"The last onset," and "Living with Kaposi's"

Lynch had a sense that his feature article on AIDS—which warned against panic and called for critical thinking—would be important. This was, after all, 1982, and the fear among gay men was palpable. *"It's gonna be a blockbuster,"* he wrote in his diary. So convinced was Lynch of the importance of both his article and its more scientific companion piece ("The Real Gay Epidemic: Panic and Paranoia," by Bill Lewis), that he fundraised to pay for the extra costs associated with running the two long articles together in a longer than usual issue of *The Body Politic.*

"Living with Kaposi's," published in the November 1982 issue of *The Body Politic*, provoked a barrage of letters to the editor and a storm of controversy among influential writers in the United States. The article appeared one year and five months after the U.S. Centers for Disease Control published its first brief report on what would become known as AIDS. By the fall of 1982, 625 cases had been reported in the United States and 14 in Canada. The mortality rate was shocking: 41 per cent of the total cases reported had already resulted in death. Most of those with AIDS were gay men, although hemophiliacs and heterosexuals had also contracted the syndrome.[27] Hemophiliacs in particular used blood products made from the blood of hundreds of individuals, which greatly increased their risk of contracting AIDS.

Lynch's six thousand-word article opened with the "human interest" story of his New York friend Larry Okin, who had AIDS, and revealed how Larry's lover, friends, and parents were coping with his bouts of illness. (Okin was called "Fred" in Lynch's article.) But it went on to assert that gay men must look carefully at where they were headed in their response to the epidemic. In the face of this frightening new illness, Lynch argued, gay men were in danger of relinquishing their identity and power to the medical and research establishments, without due recognition of the biases and interests of those groups. How is it that New York has "tumbled so readily and swiftly into the medicalization trap?" Lynch asked. Doctors, he charged, were attempting to define the gay community in terms of this illness; they were cloaking a moral program in medical terms. In New York, he said, panic was common and members of the gay community were busy raising money and handing it over to doctors and researchers. They were yielding to medical mediators and frenzied fundraising.

Lynch's article aroused strong emotions because it tackled AIDS from a different angle than anything previously seen. The tone of his reflections was noticeably different from the panicked voices in the gay press south of the border, especially the *New York Native*. In the same month that Lynch's article appeared in *The Body Politic*, another landmark article was published in the *New York Native*: "We Know Who We are: Two Gay Men Declare War on Promiscuity," by Michael Callen and Richard Berkowitz. Indeed, the two papers "hit the stands in New York, as though by prearrangement, the same day," Nathan Fain observed in *The Advocate*.[28] In "We Know Who We Are," the authors concluded that "there is no mutant virus" and instead blamed their own promiscuity for the fact that they had contracted AIDS. "We know who we are and we know why we're sick."

A half-year before, in April 1982, in an article in *The Advocate* about Gay-Related Immunodeficiency (GRID, an early name for AIDS), Fain had written, "One word is like a hand grenade in the whole affair: promiscuity."[29] A key and persistent problem in discussions about AIDS would be the confusion of statistical probability with moral judgement.

Lynch's approach might have gained a certain distance simply because he lived in Toronto—or at least not in New York, which was already at the centre of the emerging AIDS maelstrom. When he wrote the article, Toronto had seen only two cases of AIDS, and Canada as a whole fourteen, while the largest proportion of the more than six hundred cases south of border were from New York City. Canada would lag about two years behind the United States in the progress of the epidemic: the Gay Men's Health Crisis was founded in New York in 1981; it would be 1983 before a similar organization, the AIDS Committee of Toronto, emerged in Ontario's capital city.

In his article Lynch proposed two explanations for what had been happening. Deep within gay men, he said, there "lingered a readiness to find ourselves guilty. We were ripe to embrace a viral infection as a moral punishment. The media nourished this readiness but did not create it." But as well, when faced with illness, gay men tended to react by distancing themselves and by turning to doctors rather than looking to their gay community for help. "We yielded our own power to deal creatively with all aspects of our life, including dying."

Lynch's prime concern was the "equation that gay equals pathology," and he called for an all-out campaign to counter that tendency. "We can only protest the inaccuracy and inhumanity of the anti-sexual straight press, but we can demand that the gay press give a fuller human picture of support groups and first-person experiences." Gays needed to challenge the medical profession, to establish their own priorities, and any money raised should follow those priorities. Gay activists should get "a much fuller picture of the political terrain among researchers" before contributing to cancer research. They should find out what funds were available from other sources. As a first priority they should "spend money on our gay brothers who need expensive medical care." Second, they should carry on the media campaign; and, third, make sure that any money available was being tapped for the necessary research. To challenge the drift into medicalization, Lynch suggested that they might want to demand gay space in hospitals. They would "surely want institutional recognition of our friends and lovers on a par with recognition of our families. We must widen our efforts at founding gay hospices and other forms of outpatient care."

Lynch's article was praised by the *Bay Area Reporter*, a San Francisco gay publication, but denounced by leading U.S. AIDS writers such as Dr. Lawrence Mass, who was writing for the *New York Native*, and Dr. Dan Williams, who had been quoted in the gay and straight press. They took Lynch to task for not urging gay men to limit the number of their sexual partners, a criticism echoed by New York activist Michael Callen, whose letter to *The Body Politic* stated: "We cannot allow our knee-jerk defensiveness to delay urgently needed, rational discussion about the health hazards of promiscuity."

These were early days and HIV (human immunodeficiency virus, widely accepted as the cause of AIDS) had not yet been identified, but many doctors and scientists were already assuming that AIDS was caused by an infectious agent, spread through sexual contact. By not denouncing "promiscuity" as the "cause" of AIDS—indeed, in his companion piece Lewis referred to promiscuity as a factor that "knits together the social fabric of the gay male community"—Lynch and Lewis were swimming against the tide. Replying to a stinging letter from Vancouver's Dr. Brian Willoughby, Lynch wrote: "I have never, as Dr. Willoughby suggests, said that gay men should be promiscuous. I do believe, however, that much of what we now know as gay community and gay political power came about as a result of our struggle to make physical and emotional contacts with one another."

Meanwhile, in his article, microbiologist Lewis struggled to make the point that blaming promiscuity was confusing a statistical phenomenon—the more partners, the higher the risk of contracting AIDS—with a judgmental one. "Having only a moderate number of sexual partners," he noted, "is no guarantee that AIDS will be avoided."

Theoretically, Canada gained a certain advantage given that the emerging AIDS epidemic was two years behind that in the United States. People in Canada had time to prepare for the onslaught, time to think about ways of stemming the tide. But in practical terms, there was almost no preparation carried out in medical institutions and public health departments. For a time there was also a widespread belief that somehow the mysterious new illness was geographically specific—people became infected only in New York and

San Francisco. The more astute members of the medical/scientific profession could see the parallels with hepatitis B—"There is, in fact, a striking resemblance to hepatitis B virus infection," Bill Lewis wrote in his November 1982 *Body Politic* article. The observation gave Canadians good reason to worry, because it meant living in Canada was no protection. There would be no comfort in geography.

The Lynch article finished with a rallying cry that was prophetic:

> The organized gay community across North America needs to be preparing for the "health crisis" onset when it leaves Manhattan, as it has already begun to do. Surely we must, as a community, continue to improve our educational referral efforts. As in gay health care over the past decade, our intent must not be to frighten or to moralize, but to inform and to care.

But there was more to it as well:

> As gay individuals we must come to see death and dying not as opposed to life, but rather as a part of living. In short, we must make dying gay—in our own terms. Morbid? Not at all. The only morbidity lies in turning our backs on our ill or dying friends, or abandoning them to die straight deaths within alien families or institutions. As a community, we must develop caring rituals not just as a support for weakness but as a way to make weakness a source of strength. . . .
>
> The thrust of gay liberation, even if the term does feel nostalgic in 1982, remains that we make our own lives. That we do not sign ourselves over to the panic-mongering journalists and doctors . . . the coming months of 1983 will show whether we will acquiesce to the physicians and the press. The choice is ours.

two

BLOOD AND STIGMA

STEW NEWTON WAS busy at his typewriter at the beginning of 1983, composing warnings about the threat of "highly contagious" AIDS. His cluttered homemade flyers featured much use of capitalization, underlining, bold type, and exclamation marks, and he affixed his sprawling signature to each one.

Newton, a jewellery store owner, was the self-described chair of a group he called Positive Parents of Ontario, and the scaremongering flyers were being distributed around the city. His target was homosexuals and their "supporters," who, for him, included everyone from members of the New Democratic Party and left-wing Toronto school trustees to Prime Minister Pierre Trudeau. "There is something WRONG with a charter of RIGHTS that SUBJUGATES HETEROSEXUALS AND LIBERATES HOMOSEXUALS/criminals," Newton declared.[1] Homosexuals are the major carriers of AIDS, and victims "must be isolated now," he instructed. Urging the inspection of gay restaurants and taverns, he demanded that signs be posted in those establishments to warn clients of "the possible hazards" of eating or drinking there. Gay bathhouses should also be closed, and gay men should be publicly advised not to donate blood, lest AIDS spread into the blood supply. "Do you want homosexuals, lesbians and the homosexual N.D.P. caucus telling your police how to do their job?"

Newton, a friend of evangelist Rev. Ken Campbell, had been agitating about the "homosexual influence" in Toronto since 1980, when he organized a "pro-family" rally at City Hall. In 1981 his persistent attempts to discredit homosexuals were the subject of a September 21 protest by GLARE (Gay Liberation Against the Right Everywhere), a briefly constituted group that had coalesced after the February 1981 bathhouse raids.

Newton was so worked up about AIDS that he also fired off letters to various officials. On January 24, 1983, he wrote to Dr. A.S. (Sandy) Macpherson, Toronto's medical officer of health, advising him that all employees of "homosexually-operated businesses" should undergo "immediate health inspections" to determine if they are "A.I.D.S. carriers." When his demands went unmet, Newton charged that Toronto's chief health officer "refuses" to act. William Cardiff, the head of the Canadian Red Cross, also received a letter from Newton.

Newton's campaign was clearly hate-mongering, but he launched it into a vacuum. Neither the city nor the province had any plans underway as yet to deal with the arrival of AIDS. Nor had there yet been any gay community organizing in response to the epidemic—although Newton's homophobic campaign soon helped to spark one.

An estimated fifty thousand gay men lived in Toronto, and some of them, particularly those who travelled to the United States and had friends there, were starting to get very worried.[2] Harvey Hamburg was one of them. In the summer of 1982 Hamburg, a lawyer active with the Gay Community Appeal, had made a short trip to New York, where he met a man named Stuart on the street.[3] "He was a Jewish guy like myself," Hamburg later said. He enjoyed the encounter, and the two men made plans to get together again the next time Hamburg was in New York. But when that trip came about, Stuart didn't call. The mystery was solved when Hamburg was back in Toronto and Stuart phoned, explaining that he had lost the slip of paper with Hamburg's New York number. Some time later, before he headed out on yet another trip to New York, Hamburg telephoned Stuart. The line was out of service. In New York Hamburg went to the place where Stuart had been living, in Greenwich Village, and slipped a note under the door. A few days after he got back to Toronto, he received a letter. It was from Stuart's mother. Stuart was dead.

Robert Wallace, a professor in the drama department at York University in Toronto, said that he was "ambivalent" about the AIDS situation until he went to San Francisco in early 1983. "I had a friend, Tony Barnacot, who was a nurse there," Wallace said. "They already had AIDS wings in hospitals, and he told me stories that turned my head." But in those early days, there was also resistance to organizing to fight AIDS, Wallace explained. "A lot of people were afraid that AIDS was just another club to beat us down—not just activists but people on the streets and in the bars. They said we won't let this affect us, it's just another threat to our independent burgeoning sexuality."

Michael Lynch began the new year by visiting San Rafael, in Marin County, California. His former wife Gail and her lover, performance artist Pat Bond, lived there, and he and Stefan had gone to spend Christmas with them. Gail and Pat Bond had met through Lynch in 1979, when he brought Bond to Toronto for a benefit performance. Bond was known for her performances as Gertrude Stein and Lorena Hickok, Eleanor Roosevelt's lover. Her career took off after she appeared in *The Word Is Out: Stories of Some of Our Lives*, a 1978 documentary about gays and lesbians. Gail had moved to California in November 1980 to live with Bond. At first Stefan stayed in Toronto and spent the school year with his father and holidays with his mother. In the summer of 1984 the pattern was reversed, and he went to attend school in San Rafael.

New Year's Eve, December 31, 1982, found Lynch in a reflective mood: *"Look ahead? Impossible, just impossible. Look back? Easy, if not easy."* In the previous year his mother had died, Larry had died. He had sold the Roehampton house and bought a new one. He experienced a visit from his brother Pat *("& all it represented")*. He had broken up with one man and met another. He had *"repaired a hernia, lost weight, gained weight . . . dinner with Jane Rule, meeting Foucault, Christmas Eve with Robert Duncan."* A particularly memorable event had been "Wilde '82"—the first-ever international Lesbian and Gay History Conference, hosted by the Canadian Gay Archives and commemorating the one-hundredth anniversary of Oscar Wilde's famous North American tour. It was held at the end of June at Ryerson Polytechnic Institute in Toronto. Lynch had, he noted, begun *"teaching in a tie and chinos."* He had turned thirty-eight, designed a new house, and had a "rapprochement" with old friend Bill Lewis—they had lived together at Roehampton for three years before going their separate ways. He had a *"New closeness with Gail & Pat. And Stefan? Nothing momentous, but everything in day-to-day love."*

Planning a new house was occupying much of Lynch's mind. He had finalized the sale of 435 Roehampton on the day that his mother died. His inheritance from her enabled him to buy and renovate, jointly with Lewis, a house at 8 Ross Street, a stone's throw from the downtown campus of the University of Toronto. It was a semi-detached, three-storey home in the heart of downtown on a street that had in recent decades been home to waves of immigrants. In contrast, 435 Roehampton was in a predominantly white, middle-class neighbourhood. When he bought the Roehampton house, it had suited a young husband and father, a beginning professor whose dream—to be a university professor with a wife and family, like his mentor Tom Whitaker—was still alive, if just barely. But as that ambition disappeared, the location no longer fit. Aside from everything else that made it unsuitable, Lynch didn't own a car and public transit to the residential neighbourhood stopped at around one in the morning. After staying out late at political meetings, *Body Politic* production nights, or bars, he often found himself stranded downtown, facing costly taxicab rides home.

Lynch and Lewis had hired a young architect, William Woodworth, to divide 8 Ross in half, making it into a showpiece duplex. Lynch later wrote that his apartment was designed *"to keep me from living with a lover . . . A zest for isolation built this house."*

Lynch had to vacate Roehampton near the end of January, and for the following months, while Ross Street was being renovated, he and Stefan moved into 48 Simpson Avenue, in the Riverdale area just east of the Don Valley. It was a communal house rented by his *Body Politic* friends Ed Jackson, Gerald Hannon, and Robert Trow. Herb Spiers, a founding member of *The Body Politic* who had returned to the United States, was a friend of the house and kept them informed of developments in New York City. "We had another acquaintance die of AIDS recently," Spiers wrote on January 19, 1983.[4] "Actually, you may have met him. An old island person; wonderful chap, as sweet as they come. And tonight Peter Cooper told Ray

[Gray] that a former housemate of theirs has Kaposis. The bars are starting to hold benefits for GMHC [Gay Men's Health Crisis]. Half the bar receipts go to it."

In March Lynch wrote that he, who was *"announcing myself as the great defender of the role of promiscuity in the homo community,"* was bored with sex. And he declared himself determined to cease doing journalistic writing, especially in the pages of *The Body Politic*. His article "This Seeing the Sick Endears Them," about the AIDS death of his New York friend Larry Okin, had just been published there. The article concluded with a passage about how he and Larry's lover danced one night, and:

> with a furious rage against our loss, brought Larry back to life between us on the dance floor, electrified our bodies with an energy that could only have been his legacy entering into us as it departed from his hardy-handsome mould. A death dance, we found, is no mild, pallidly mournful mime, but a vigorous rout, a transfer of power from the dead to the living. . . . How much more powerful than the myths of transfiguration or eternal life is the charged new life of friends who have experienced loss together, who have felt themselves the recipients of their dead friend's liveliest gifts.[5]

Lynch did refrain from journalism during the rest of the year—although he wrote letters to other publications.[6] Still, after visiting New York in early March, he was already musing in his diary about organizing *"an AIDS helper group in T.O."*

Self-help: informing Toronto's gay community

The Toronto group Gays in Health Care (GHC) was beginning to wonder if it shouldn't be more active sharing information about both AIDS and hepatitis B. The hepatitis B vaccine had been licensed for use in Canada in late 1982, and microbiologist Bill Lewis, who was on the Ontario Advisory Committee on the vaccine, was pushing to have at least 10 per cent of the available vaccine set aside for gay men, the province's largest at-risk group. But some committee members argued that the vaccine should be available only to those at risk "through no fault of their own"—meaning health-care workers, who would be prone to contract the virus through accidental contact with contaminated blood, in contrast to gay men (the main risk factor was multiple sex partners) and injection drug users who shared needles.[7]

Through its members, the GHC had a loose association with the Bay Area Physicians for Human Rights. Several GHC members attended BAPHR meetings and received its newsletter, the *BAPHRON*. The February issue of that newsletter declared that because of AIDS the gay community was "in the midst of the most serious health crisis we have known." It noted that 25 per cent of AIDS cases had occurred in heterosexuals, but argued that "as a gay physicians group we must be on the forefront."

By March, Gays in Health Care had joined with Hassle Free Clinic to begin making plans for a public forum on AIDS and hepatitis B to be held at Ryerson Polytechnical in April—the first public forum on AIDS in Toronto. The more geographically cohesive Vancouver gay community had, on March 12, already hosted its first forum on AIDS, held at the West End Community Centre. That forum brought in the president of New York's Gay Men's Health Crisis, Paul Popham, as a featured speaker, and among the questioners from the audience was Gaetan Dugas, the Québécois flight attendant subsequently labelled "Patient Zero," as if he had spread AIDS through North America. AIDS Vancouver was born out of that first forum.[8]

Bill Lewis submitted a rough draft of a pamphlet on AIDS, prepared jointly with Hassle Free Clinic for the upcoming Toronto forum, in the GHC's March/April newsletter.[9] The GHC newsletter also reprinted a statement from the Research and Scientific Affairs Committee and Education Committee of the Association of American Physicians for Human Rights (AAPHR) on "AIDS and Healthful Gay Male Sexual Activity." The two-page statement outlined the general symptoms of AIDS and recommended two main steps for reducing risks. The first step was for a man to reduce the number of different men he had sex with—"and particularly with those men who also have many different sexual partners." The second step was to not inject illegal drugs and to avoid sexual contact with IV drug users. The newsletter also suggested that gay men "reduce" a number of other factors: one-time encounters with anonymous partners and/or group sex; oral-anal contact ("rimming"); fisting (both giving and receiving); active or passive rectal intercourse (use of condoms may be helpful, it said); and fecal contamination (scat). The Southern California Physicians for Human Rights group had begun recommending condoms in November 1982 "to decrease the loading of viruses which may be indicated in the syndrome."[10] No precedent existed for the use of condoms in gay sexual encounters to *prevent* disease, because, as Hassle Free Clinic counsellor Robert Trow later noted, for some time gay men had been used to straightforward, effective medical treatment for sexually transmitted diseases (STDs).

The AAPHR statement was providing advice similar to that being given in other U.S. publications. The GHC, however, added a note stressing that the statement did not represent the views of the GHC and that several members felt it to be "premature, alarmist and without substantiation." The newsletter continued: "It is the feeling of this editor that it is the responsibility of Gay Health Care workers to circulate only substantiated facts to the community. . . . Any practice to the contrary will only propagate within our own community the same detrimental prejudices which are already facing us from other groups who wish to undermine our lifestyles."

The first half of 1983 was a particularly tense time for Toronto's gay activists as, in the face of a possible epidemic, they balanced different aspects of community interests. Gay leaders like Lynch and Lewis, in their November 1982 *Body Politic* features, had already taken a strong stand against panic. Yet Lewis, especially after attending a March 1983 AIDS conference at New York University's medical school, was clearly becoming more concerned about the emerging epidemic. According to a study presented at the conference by researcher Michael Marmor, gay men who engaged in anal intercourse with numerous partners had eleven times the risk of developing Kaposi's sarcoma. "Physicians should tell homosexual patients to use condoms not only when they have sex with gay men, who are at high risk of Kaposi's, but all sex partners," Dr. Marmor said. Dr. James Curran, head of an AIDS task force set up by the Centers for Disease Control, told the conference that more than twelve hundred AIDS cases had been reported in the United States and the tally was increasing weekly. The total number included twelve hemophiliacs and twenty children, he said.[11]

In an April article in *The Body Politic*, Lewis acknowledged that "the situation is more serious than I had thought six months ago." Promiscuity did not cause AIDS, he stressed, but as with any sexually transmitted disease, the risk of contracting AIDS was greater the more sexual partners one had. "If we choose to decrease the number of sexual partners we have, it should have the effect of reducing possible exposure to the infectious agent that causes AIDS. How large that reduction in risk will be depends on the percentage of infected men in any particular location." Lewis also stressed that some AIDS patients had very few contacts. He concluded: "The challenge to us now is not only to provide information and support for those at risk and those who are ill. Our challenge is also to anticipate and counter our enemies' exploitation of our newest vulnerability." Lewis's informative and thoughtful article, meanwhile, was topped with a headline —"AIDS: Discounting the Promiscuity Theory"—which appeared to be intended more to calm nerves than to accurately represent the text.

In the June issue of the newsmagazine, Richard Summerbell, a *Body Politic* regular and University of Toronto professor of mycology, took issue with Lewis's arguments.

> From a medical point of view, Bill Lewis's article . . . was a very good one. However, Lewis's comments on promiscuity struck me as overly optimistic . . . one thing we can be assured of is that some kinds of gay sex are among the easiest known modes of human disease transmission. Doctors have told us that we may make direct contact with the bloodstream by means of "minute cuts and abrasions during anal sex," while the intestinal-oral contact in rimming has given us many of our hepatitis A and parasite problems. . . . All that is required of us, in our "new sexual ethic," is that we have sex in a way that favours us more than it favours our diseases.

Psychiatrist Stephen Atkinson, a founder of Toronto's GHC and participant in early organizing around AIDS, saw the tensions in the community as being "between the 'conservatives,' who were safety-conscious, and the 'politicals,' who said they were trying to reduce panic." He believed the "politicals" were acutely aware of how the disease "could be used against us, and wanted the gay community not to retreat in any way from the more radical, forthright, 'we're OK, dammit' message since Stonewall." Atkinson saw himself as a moderate on these questions. He believed that there was very good reason for gays, including himself, to change their behaviour based on the evidence at hand. He also thought, as he had some for some time, "that the 'political' point of view seemed wedded to the idea of promiscuity as liberation from heterosexist oppressive norms."

The gay community and the Canadian Red Cross Society

In the first few months of 1983 the response to AIDS began to focus in on the matter of blood donations. In Toronto, for one thing, the flyers being distributed by Positive Parents were screaming out that homosexuals were the major carriers of AIDS and that AIDS was transmissible through blood transfusions. The risk to the blood supply had also received some attention in the press. "AIDS: Blood Bank's Hidden Bomb," by Terry Murray, had been published in the Dec. 28, 1982 issue of *The Medical Post*. A Montreal study had found that 70 per cent of hemophiliacs had an immune deficiency similar to that found in AIDS. In January, under the headline "Killer Disease Linked to Blood: Evidence Points to Contagious Agent in Mysterious Illness," an article quoted Dr. Jay Keystone of the Toronto General Hospital noting that "everything points to a transmissible agent."[12] In the United States the integrity of the blood supply had already been identified as an important and potentially explosive issue, and the Centers for Disease Control set up a meeting in January to discuss blood-donor policies. Dr. Curran of the CDC's AIDS task force expressed concern that the issue of restricting donors versus cleaning up blood would cause division.

Early in the year, prompted by Stew Newton's flyer campaign, Ed Jackson of *The Body Politic* was researching an article and contacted the Canadian Red Cross Society for a comment.[13] It would be only one of many meetings of a gay activist with the Red Cross over the next long while as their concerns began to mesh. And it was relatively convenient to meet with the Red Cross Society officials. The Society's national offices were on Wellesley Street between Jarvis and Church streets, close to Toronto's gay ghetto. The Hassle Free Clinic was close too, just around the corner on Church Street, not far from the 519 Community Centre.

By March 1983 Jackson was reporting in *The Body Politic*, "The Canadian Red Cross Society, the agency responsible for virtually all blood collection in this country, has resisted pressure from at least one anti-gay organization to ban blood donations from homosexuals." As of February 7, there were twenty-six cases with AIDS-like symptoms reported in Canada. Jackson quoted a federal official who stated that sixteen of the cases involved gay men, ten of whom had already died. He reported that there was "a complete lack of medical evidence" to support the Positive Parents' claims.[14] Dr. John Derrick of the Red Cross said "that if evidence eventually became clear that blood transfusions and AIDS transmission are related, it would be necessary to institute stricter screening of blood donors. At such time, the Red Cross would follow the stated American policy of going to leaders of the gay community for help in conveying information to potential donors."

The meeting that the U.S. Centers for Disease Control had called for January 4, 1983, was attended by representatives of the gay community, the American Red Cross, and federal health agencies. Dr. Curran had outlined a number of approaches to screening blood, including screening for hepatitis B core antigen. The virus linked to AIDS had not yet been identified, but hepatitis B displayed similar transmission patterns, so that screening for hepatitis B could effectively mean screening for the agent causing AIDS. "But I think the best thing politically for the gay community," he said, "would be to withhold giving blood voluntarily, to take the political initiative. . . . The thing is, people are dying. The medical problem is more important than the civil rights issues."[15] The U.S. gay leadership, however, proposed another course: screen blood, not donors, and protect the rights of gay citizens.

Toronto soon faced the same dilemma. At the beginning of March, the Canadian Hemophilia Society released a recommendation urging people who might be at risk for AIDS not to donate blood.

On Friday, March 4, the U.S. assistant secretary of health, Edward Brandt, recommended to volunteer blood collection agencies that they request donors from groups at high risk of developing AIDS to refrain from donating blood. On March 8 a *Medical Post* article written by Terry Murray, a key early reporter on AIDS in Canada, appeared over the headline "AIDS: Come out of Closet, Donors Urged." That same day Dr. Derrick contacted Jackson "with reference to initiating a means of communication with Canadian homosexuals concerning the CRC position on blood-donor screening."[16] In the course of their conversation, Jackson told Derrick that Gays in Health Care and Hassle Free Clinic were together preparing a pamphlet on AIDS.

Later, in his draft statement prepared for testifying before the Commission of Inquiry on the Blood System in Canada (the Krever Commission), Jackson would report about that time: "I felt that Dr. Derrick was pleasant and courteous but did not understand the nature of the gay community. I explained to him that the gay community was not organized in the sense of having a recognized leadership or any structure. I said that there was no guarantee of reaching every member of the gay community because many gay people are not open about their sexuality."[17]

Two days later, the Red Cross issued a press release, and *The Globe and Mail*, in its bulldog (early evening) edition, duly reported that all homosexuals, along with drug abusers and Haitians, were being asked not to donate blood. Alarmed at this story, Jackson called Dr. Derrick at home, and Derrick called the *Globe* to "clarify" that only certain homosexuals should refrain. Hence, between editions the paper changed the opening of the story from "The Canadian Red Cross is asking homosexuals, drug abusers and Haitians not to give blood" to "The Canadian Red Cross is advising promiscuous male homosexuals, drug abusers and Haitians . . ." Dr. Derrick was quoted in the later edition as saying, "Sexual transmission is related to the high degree of promiscuity in the male. Active male homosexuals or bisexuals with multiple partners would be the classification we'd be most concerned about."[18]

The debate over who should refrain from donating blood underscored a charged political issue—concern about an entire group being stigmatized—that would lead to conflict between the Red

Cross and representatives of Toronto's gay community later in 1983. The issue had been taken up earlier by the National Gay Task Force in the United States. An NGTF press release dated January 10 decried the "sheer impracticability" of a voluntary abstention approach, while pointing to greater issues. "Such a policy is reminiscent of miscegenation blood laws that divided black blood from white," it noted. (During the Second World War the U.S. War Department had issued a directive that blood taken from white donors should be segregated from the blood of Black donors. The pioneering Black doctor Charles Drew, who had set up the first U.S. blood bank, resigned in protest as project director for the American Red Cross.)

Jackson convened a group of ten men, including himself, to respond to the Red Cross request about disseminating information on blood donation warnings. Lynch was at the Saturday, March 12, meeting, along with Robert Trow of Hassle Free Clinic and a number of Gays in Health Care regulars—Dr. Randy Coates, Dr. Stan Read, Bill Lewis, and Dr. Don Briggs—as well as Dr. Jack Fowler, social worker David Kelley, and archivist Alan Miller, author of the first bibliography of gays and AIDS.[19] "At first the consensus seemed to be that it was best to ask all gay people to refrain from giving blood. Resistance to this began to grow," the meeting minutes stated. Lynch, helped by Trow, subsequently drew up a document, "AIDS and the Canadian Gay Male Community: Contexts and Issues," which summarized the March 12 discussion for consideration at a subsequent meeting scheduled for March 22.[20] The document suggested that the situation in Canada was much like that in New York two years earlier. Canada so far had relatively few confirmed cases, "but, given the history of AIDS, we should expect a significant rate of increase in its incidence here in the coming months."

As Lynch and Trow pointed out, the task of minimizing panic, misunderstanding, and stigmatization in a homophobic and racist society was a difficult one. "The primary victims—gay men, Haitians, certain users of recreational drugs—have been painted as victimizers. Minimizing the spread of AIDS to lower-risk groups has sometimes taken precedence over minimizing its spread among the high-risk (but socially "undesirable") groups—as the Red Cross Society's actions may well demonstrate."

That observation would prove to be an accurate assessment of much of the official Canadian response to AIDS—although the assumption that hemophiliacs were among those at low risk would prove terribly wrong. As it turned out, hemophiliacs were not "lower risk" than homosexuals. According to the Canadian Hemophilia Society, about 90 per cent of some eight hundred Canadians who suffered from severe hemophilia A, the most common type of severe hemophilia, were infected with HIV before blood and blood products were made safe. Of the total number of Canadians with hemophilia (mild, moderate, and severe), about 30 to 35 per cent were infected with HIV.[21]

But it was also true that the gay community was itself just beginning to make an effort to provide information to prevent the spread of AIDS in its own community, or to press the city's Public Health Department in that direction. After all, so far only a couple of dozen cases of AIDS had been identified in all of Canada. As well, the main recommendation to reduce risk was to make changes in sexual behaviour—reduce the number of sexual partners, be monogamous, or refrain from sex altogether. (Safer sex through condom use was not yet being widely advocated.) Toronto's gay community had fought hard to defend its right to sexuality, and it would be hard pressed to advocate such measures. The gay leaders were also continuing to make a conscious effort to avoid the panic-driven, self-flagellating approach to change advocated south of the border.

The Making of the AIDS Committee

The document "AIDS and the Canadian Gay Male Community" explored important issues. Will a request that all homosexuals refrain from donating blood "maximize public misunderstanding," leading to the belief that all gay men are a danger to everyone else's health? How effective is it to ask those who are ill or have symptoms to refrain from donating blood when there appears to be a carrier state in AIDS? Is the volunteer Canadian blood collection system safer than the U.S. system, which includes paid donors? The document ended with two crucial points for anyone interested in organizing around the issues: "Should the gay community begin organizing for an AIDS task force, to be able to speak for the community on such occasions as that provided recently by the Red Cross and the *Globe*? Should the community organize both an AIDS-patient Support Group? and perhaps a more general counselling program for dealing with critical health issues, as through the Counselling Centre?"

The document emphasized creating a new organization to speak for the community and to help those already sick—and did not emphasize preventing the spread of AIDS. That task would be taken up soon, but certainly any effort to change sexual behaviour would be complicated. Lynch, for example, had been in New York on the weekend before he met with the other men to formulate a response to the Red Cross. He had gone to visit Bruce Schentes, whose lover Larry Okin had died of AIDS, and he "crunched into tears" upon visiting their apartment for the first time since Larry's death. Later in the evening, after that loaded and emotional experience, he went to The Saint, the city's premiere gay disco. It was the most up-to-date technically and artistically of the bars. "It was the ne plus ultra . . . like heaven, magical, huge in scale, fun, well organized and run, totally fabulous," as Spiers described it later. At the disco, Lynch picked up *"a cute 20ish looking trick lad . . . as we were fucking and cuddling (both done very well by each) I thought continually about AIDS."*

Haitians in Montreal also organized in response to the Red Cross statement. On March 11, a group of seven Haitian organizations, including the Association of Haitian Doctors Abroad, issued a release noting that no scientific evidence supported the statement that the Haitian community was a population at risk and that no cause and effect could be established between any national group and a non-hereditary pathological condition. "The media's sensationalistic treatment of this issue has created a state of panic in the Haitian Community," the release continued, "and has provoked both groups and individuals to react irrationally toward this ethnic minority which has been stigmatized indiscriminately and in the absence of conclusive evidence."[22]

In a *Medical Post* article about the Haitian protest and Red Cross initiatives, Jackson commented: "We'd be more concerned about asking why it is that no government or board of health has spent a cent on getting information out to the gay community about the dangers of AIDS. Why isn't one of the highest risk groups being informed about the dangers rather than protecting a minuscule, low risk group like hemophiliacs?"[23] The Toronto Board of Health had just commissioned its first report on AIDS, but it was basically an information sheet on the illness.[24]

Jackson's "group of ten" convened again on March 22, this time without Fowler and Kelley, but with Harvey Hamburg, the lawyer who worked with the Gay Community Appeal. The group decided not to make a public statement about blood donations. If asked, they agreed to tell the media that gay medical and community leaders "quietly endorse a Red Cross policy that, until a blood-screening process to detect AIDS is established, gay men refrain from giving blood 'because of what we don't know.'"

The group also made a decision to set up an "interim structure," preliminary to organizing an ongoing AIDS committee, in order to be able to respond to those who would attend the Ryerson forum on AIDS, to be held on April 5. Hassle Free Clinic's Trow reported that he had approached the local Board of Health about funding for the pamphlet on AIDS that he and Lewis were developing. The pamphlet would now include a section on blood donations, stressing the theme of minimizing the spread of disease.

Flyers for the Ryerson event gave top billing to hepatitis B ("Is your health in danger? Come find out about hepatitis B and AIDS"), while an advertisement in the April issue of *The Body Politic* gave AIDS the top spot. In all, about three hundred people were attracted to the GHC forum. The speakers included doctors Randy Coates and Stan Read, and Bill Lewis. *"An orderly and tame, intelligent and sex positive AIDS/HPB meeting tonight, at which Billy spoke on AIDS—my first time, actually, hearing him speak,"* Lynch wrote. Fifty-two men who attended the Ryerson meeting signed papers saying they were willing to participate in the formation of a new organization, which would be something "like the Right To Privacy Committee, to respond to this crisis as a lesbian/gay community organization but . . . not restricted to gays, " said Karsten Kossmann, who became the first executive director of the new organization.[25]

For the next couple of months or more—until the end of June, when a much larger community meeting about AIDS was held—a great deal of energy went into organizing what was then referred to as the Toronto AIDS Committee. Talks were also continuing with the Red Cross Society. On April 8, Jackson, Read, Coates, and Trow met with Red Cross representatives to outline their concerns about the stigmatization of gay men. They also showed the Red Cross a draft of the AIDS pamphlet that Lewis and Trow were still working on. The draft included a paragraph on the Red Cross request that groups at high risk of contracting AIDS refrain from donating blood.[26]

Two weeks after the April 5 Ryerson meeting, Lynch, Jackson, Hamburg, Atkinson, Lewis, and Trow met to identify areas that needed work around AIDS. They were all veteran activists and organizers, and saw the merit of presenting a framework to the larger group. On April 26, Trow outlined the plan to about forty-five people who attended a planning meeting at the 519 Church Street Community Centre.

Some participants were disgruntled because the organizers had already set up an agenda—when the purpose of the meeting was purportedly to begin a process of defining a structure. But the six subcommittees envisioned by the organizers were established: education, support, political action/fundraising, medical issues, media, and a subcommittee to liaise with other AIDS organizations and produce a list of medical and social referrals. The temporary centre for the new organization was at the men's section of Hassle Free Clinic, where Trow worked. The Toronto AIDS Committee was, in effect, born, although the organizers did not formally announce its birth for over two months. The members involved in fundraising soon took steps to apply for a $62,000 federal government grant, through an Employment Development Program, to fund "community education around AIDS."[27]

For the members of this new group, the biggest questions revolved around the noticeable reluctance of the established institutions and authorities to take action. Why were local boards of health taking absolutely no initiative in distributing information about the disease to the gay community and other groups at risk, including the Haitians? Why were the provincial and federal governments not acting as quickly as possible to fund primary research on AIDS? Why, Ed Jackson asked in a *Body Politic* editorial, were the ministers of health being utterly silent about a disease that had "already killed more people than swine flu, toxic shock and Legionnaire's disease combined?" Even worse, crucial scientific information was being held back. At the March AIDS conference in New York, two researchers had been booed for refusing to divulge study findings before publication. "The medical establishment encourages secrecy, fierce competition for funding and individual career-building over speedy solutions to health problems," Jackson wrote. "Could that information be helping to save lives right now?"[28]

"Fighting for Our Lives": representation and the Denver Principles

At the end of April, en route to Dunn to visit Lynch's dying grandmother, Lynch and Stefan went to New York for the weekend. Stefan was excited about getting to know the city. Father and son spent Saturday afternoon with Larry Okin's grieving parents. They all had lunch together and then went to a street fair hosted by the Chelsea Gay Association. Lynch found it strange to be there on the streets with Okin's parents, "the survivors," as they walked through the crowd being solicited to contribute to the fight against AIDS. That evening, April 30, Lynch, Stefan, Spiers, and Jackson (who was also in the city) were four of the 17,600 who attended the Ringling Bros. and Barnum & Bailey AIDS benefit circus at Madison Square Gardens, put on by Gay Men's Health Crisis. The circus event reportedly raised $250,000, but Lynch was not impressed. He *"felt a distance, a cold quality, as opposed to a real gay event."* Later, at The Saint, he danced, overdosed on the drug THC, and had hallucinations. He *"went to the balcony and jo'd, allowing no mucosal contact."* (This was the first suggestion in his diary that he was heeding any of the recommended precautions about sexual contact.)

The AIDS epidemic was gathering force and causing increasing alarm in gay communities in the United States. More than 1,400 people had been diagnosed in the United States, and the numbers were rising rapidly. Candlelight vigils to protest government inaction were held in major U.S. cities on Monday, May 2. About nine thousand gays and lesbians took part in a candlelight march in New York, and ten thousand marched in San Francisco. "Our president doesn't seem to know AIDS exists," activist Mark Feldman told the San Francisco crowd. "He is spending more money on the paint to put the American flag on his missiles than he's spending on AIDS."[29] (Feldman died of AIDS a month later.)

Lynch's friend Robert Reinhard was at the San Francisco vigil and reported to Lynch and Lewis that the San Franciscans were confused and uncertain. New problems were being generated every week by the AIDS crisis, he said—"new fears, new social practices and theories." The U.S. experience was, again, more heightened— more advanced in time—than was the case in Canada.

> On the one hand, you hear horrible stories of panic and disintegration of gay social relationships, and on the other heightened awareness and the formation of new social ties and institutions which are sensitive to the needs of people who have AIDS, their friends, and others. Our candlelight march last week was very moving and I think, as a symbolic demonstration, did a lot to put things in perspective. People have definitely changed their sexual behaviour patterns and look suspiciously on potential partners so that in those instances where someone might go home with a new person, the lovers feel a threat of contagion mixed in with their erotic pleasure taking. . . . I hope we will all examine the consequences to ourselves of giving over our sexual freedom in the face of conservative social pressure and scientific uncertainty.[30]

In Canada a few days later, the federal government announced an Ad Hoc Task Force on AIDS, to be chaired by Alastair Clayton, director-general of Health Canada's Laboratory Centre for Disease Control. Lynch and others were quick to protest the task force's complete lack of representatives from the risk groups. Clayton said it would not be appropriate to include interest groups in discussions of such a highly technical and scientific nature.[31]

On June 1, the province of Ontario followed suit with its own six-member committee, which was to advise the government on medical service needs, essentially to look out for the interests of health-care professionals. Asked if the gay community would be represented on this group, Ontario Health Minister Larry Grossman replied, "We have an advisory committee on cancer and we don't have cancer victims on it."[32]

The gay community's immediate demand for representation on official AIDS bodies is striking. Indeed, its eventual success in gaining such representation paved the way for other "patient groups" and transformed medical politics. The demand for representation sprang directly from the democratic politics of gay liberation, which insisted that the only people who could speak about homosexuality were homosexuals. "There are no experts on peoples' lives except those people themselves," as Spiers put it. But the demand was also influenced by the community's close links with the women's health movement, especially around the abortion rights issue. In the health field feminists were insisting not just on having more women doctors, but also on having lay women represent themselves.

Events were now rapidly unfolding—and the focus of concern, the way in which AIDS was being represented, was shifting just as quickly. In early June 1983 the term "People With AIDS" came into common currency at a Denver health-care conference. The event, attended by more than 375 people, mostly health professionals, was the Fifth National Lesbian/Gay Health Conference, and included the Second National Forum on AIDS and the First National American Association of Physicians for Human Rights Symposium.

At one conference session a small group of fourteen people with AIDS held up a banner stating: "Fighting for our lives." The attendance of people with AIDS at the Denver conference "brought a new dimension to what might otherwise have been a dry and impersonal affair," reported the *New York Native*.[33] "In fact, they offered a new way of understanding, of integrating scientific data with emotional realities." The *New York Native* writer saw the presence of "People With AIDS" as "a moving reminder" of the true role of health-care providers: to serve people, "whether the treatment is AIDS or anything else." People living with AIDS (PWAS) were "demanding to be their own advocates" and insisting "on their right to control their lives, their healing and their own destinies."

The "Denver Principles," developed by PWAS at that conference, read in part: "We condemn attempts to label us 'victims,' which implies defeat, and we are only occasionally 'patients,' which implies passivity, helplessness, and dependence on the care of others." One of the PWAS at the Denver conference was New Yorker Bob Cecchi, who would later figure in Toronto AIDS activism. Also in attendance were Dr. Richard Isaac, from Toronto's Gays in Health Care, and Halifax doctor Bob Frederickson. Later, when Frederickson testified before the Commission of Inquiry on the Blood System in Canada, he recalled the emotional response that he'd had at Denver when he realized that AIDS was definitely on its way to Canada. On his return to Halifax, the doctor went on CBC-Radio to warn people of the coming epidemic. The city's Public Health Department, however, waved aside his concern, and countered that only about 10 to 15 per cent of Halifax gays—or, it estimated, only fifteen to twenty people—would get AIDS.[34] Until 1985, neither the province of Nova Scotia nor the Halifax Public Health Department "energized" education about AIDS, the doctor testified. All of the very necessary energy to deal with the crisis came from the affected communities and from their own "devastation."[35] While governments in Canada primarily responded to AIDS by setting up advisory committees, it was the gay communities in Vancouver, Winnipeg, Toronto, Montreal, and Halifax, together with some gay and activist doctors, that were working to disseminate information about AIDS.[36]

In Toronto, throughout May and June, the various subcommittees of the new AIDS organization were busy meeting around the city. On June 9, the federal grant that the group had applied for to fund community education was approved.[37] Under the terms of the grant, the organization itself had to contribute $9,290. "It was unusual for a gay organization to get funding so fast," Jackson noted. Indeed, Karsten Kossmann, the first staff person hired, said there was controversy about the grant because of concern that by accepting government money, the committee would be inclined to restrict its operations. Lawyer Hamburg had been instrumental in obtaining the grant, and it was his last direct involvement with the committee, Kossmann noted.

Minutes of most of the early meetings were recorded and have been preserved—a testament both to the organizing abilities of the individuals involved and to their awareness of the importance of what was being created. Notable by their absence from this early work were some of the city's most seasoned gay activists, including people who had been involved in the Right to Privacy Committee.

According to Robert Wallace, who worked on the media subcommittee of the new AIDS committee, many of the old-time activists saw AIDS organizing as "unnecessary and counterproductive to the growth of the gay community." They were leery of diverting funding and attention away from gay activism and putting it into a cause which at that point still seemed to have its locus in the United States.

At the end of May Lynch returned from a flying (two-day) trip to Dunn, where he had attended the funeral of his grandmother "Mammy," his mother's mother, who had died May 27 at age ninety-seven. *"Now, really, is my chance,"* he wrote in his diary. *"The Driver women are behind me, not in front of me. Can I be true?"*

He came home in a terrible mood. No sooner had he arrived and greeted Stefan than he had to leave for an AIDS committee meeting, which he attended out of a sense of duty more than anything else. He had promised Lewis that he would help out—after all, he noted, Bill had helped him out "ages ago" by going to meetings of the Committee to Defend John Damien. Now Lynch only "half" wanted to get involved, perhaps "not even half." He sat through the meeting feeling hostile and bored—with the boredom *"so aggressively presenting itself I had to recognize the hostility."* Then he went home and was hostile to Stefan—*"hard on him. He must be eager to get to California, far far from me."*

But that May 31 meeting was a decisive one. It endorsed the new organization's official name, "AIDS Committee of Toronto," or ACT, and made a key decision to take an expansive approach. It would offer its services not just to gay patients but to everyone with AIDS, and advertise the existence of ACT through other high-risk communities.

Within a few days Lynch was feeling better about the AIDS work. At a June 9 media subcommittee meeting, he even agreed to act as media spokesperson for the AIDS Committee of Toronto. Hosted by Wallace, the meeting was also attended by Alan Miller, Ken Hutchinson, and Stephen Fontaine.[38] Lynch noted that it was his *"first such activist role in several years."* He liked the people there, he said—although except for the presence of one younger committee member the whole thing felt like a recast of the earlier days of gay activism: *"like reinventing the wheel, or at least the ball bearing."*

three
AGAINST HYSTERIA

THE EVOLVING POLITICS around AIDS led to festering disagreements in the community, and one of them involved lawyer Harvey Hamburg.

In early 1983, on one of his regular visits to New York, Hamburg had attended a Gay Men's Health Crisis meeting. Afterwards he introduced himself to Bob Cecchi, a GMHC member who went around to hospitals to visit people with AIDS, and soon after they spent a day together touring hospitals. "That was the beginning of a relationship with Bob," Hamburg said, and it would be an uneasy connection because Cecchi was sure he had AIDS. At the time there was still no test for the disease. Swollen lymph glands and a weak immune system raised red flags, while the appearance of one of the common opportunistic infections—PCP or Kaposi's sarcoma—firmed up a diagnosis. As a result, for Hamburg the new relationship was both "frightening and titillating." Cecchi invited him back to his place at the end of that first day, and they spent the night together. "I remember very distinctly putting my head down on the sheets in his bed and wondering, is this a safe thing to do?"

As a community leader and executive director of the Gay Community Appeal, Hamburg was scheduled to be one of the keynote speakers at the annual Pride Day in Toronto on June 26, held downtown on the University of Toronto campus. Keynote speakers routinely submitted a copy of their remarks in advance, and in an unusual move the Pride Day committee called Hamburg to a meeting about his speech. The problem? Hamburg's cautious approach to sex, and his advocacy of condom use. "There was some internal stuff on the Pride Day committee about whether what I was saying was anti-gay or somehow inappropriate, that I was being alarmist or those kinds of things," Hamburg said later. Indeed, a few days before Pride Day, Lynch told his diary that he was annoyed *"with Harvey Hamburg's AIDS politics."* [1]

In his speech, Hamburg told the crowd:

> For most of us, coming to accept our sexuality has involved the discovery of innumerable sexual delights. And that sex has been terrific. But for gay men, at least some of that has changed. Because of what we don't know, and because we want to live, many of us are using condoms when having anal sex, and at least for the moment, we're giving up on oral sex too, because taking lots of different people's cum might be causing us problems. But I've had some personal experience with this, and believe me, sex can still be terrific. And this message, that safe-sex is possible, has got to get through to all of us gay men. So please, spread that word and recommend it. And as you know, for many of us, casual sex has been primarily a vehicle, a way to meet men, to make the human connections that we long for. And now apparently, just in time, dating is coming back into style. You remember dating, that's where you get to know the person before. And while I'm not generally into fashions, this one could save our lives. Practising safe-sex and dating will greatly reduce the spread of AIDS, I don't know that, but that's my opinion, and I want to shout it from the rooftops, that's how concerned I am. [2]

In Lynch's view, Hamburg was simply on *"a mission to promote condoms,"* and three days later, at a community meeting on AIDS held at Jarvis Collegiate Institute, the issue came to the fore once again.

The Jarvis Collegiate meeting drew an overflow crowd of seven or eight hundred people. The high school, located at the corner of Wellesley and Jarvis streets, boasts a school auditorium that seats about 550 on the main floor, and on June 29 the place was jam-packed with people ready to hear from the "headliners": Dr. Stan Read of the Hospital For Sick Children (infectious diseases department), Lynch, and Cecchi from Gay Men's Health Crisis. Read was scheduled to provide the most up-to-date scientific understanding of AIDS, Lynch to address the politics of AIDS, and Cecchi to speak of his more personal experiences with AIDS.

The size of the crowd on a Wednesday evening took organizers by surprise, Hamburg said, although Lynch told his diary that the meeting was quiet, *"tranquil in the outer layers"*—except for Hamburg's intervention, which amounted to a *"pushing of his sex guidelines."*

Lynch's scepticism about condoms would disappear fast enough, but he wasn't the only one who was dubious. According to Robert Trow, who was still working at the Hassle Free Clinic twenty years later, the activists were aware of condoms but made "a decision not to talk about them, at the very first." They believed that emphasizing condoms would be an overreaction. Given the small number of cases up to that point in Canada, Trow said, "There was no way that gay men were going to go along with condoms."

Members of ACT's public education committee—which included Hamburg—themselves came under fire on the issue of safe sex. A pamphlet they produced for the Jarvis meeting recommended condom use for anal sex. Under a section headed "rectal sex," "Gay Sex and AIDS: Guidelines for Risk Reduction" noted:

> It isn't fair but there seems to be a definite statistical correlation between getting fucked and getting AIDS. The lining of the rectum is susceptible to tears or abrasions which you can't feel and which may last for some time. There is only one safe way of dealing with this. *Make sure that your partner is wearing a condom.* The advantage of reducing the number of your partners for this kind of sex are well worth considering. Your ass really is precious—so don't just give it to anyone.

Lionel Morton, who helped write this and other pamphlets, noted in a study of ACT's brochures that some people thought the pamphlet handed out at Jarvis was not appropriate for the Toronto audience because AIDS was not yet widespread in the city. Epidemiologist Randy Coates criticized it because he said it did not mention the best risk reduction technique of all—avoiding sex with people from New York, San Francisco, and Los Angeles.[3]

At the Jarvis meeting Cecchi spoke about the reactions of his family and friends, the situation in New York City (how, without socialized medicine many AIDS patients were being financially ruined), and how he was now handling his own sex life. Stephen Atkinson recalled that Cecchi got the safe-sex point across quite dramatically: "The part I remember is that he talked about licking armpits as a substitute for 'rimming' (anilingus, I'm not sure what lingo you're familiar with); I can't quote how he did it, but he spoke about the fact we didn't know what was safe anymore or not, and that, under those circumstances, 'I'm getting into licking armpits, you know what I mean?'—something like that, and the crowd roared."

In his speech, Lynch talked about the choices facing the gay community.[4] The community, he argued, was facing a major assault, and members must fight "against hysteria and for sanity, rationality and fact." The "don't knows" include the nature of the virus that causes AIDS "and the conditions under which it thrives," whether or not it is transmissible through saliva and semen (as well as through blood and intimate sexual contact), and whether there was a carrier phase, when it was infectious, and whether it could be resisted. A climate of such uncertainty, Lynch told the crowd, leads to three inappropriate reactions: non-medical explanations, false certitudes, and "the extremist eliminate-all-risk" solutions. He spent some time comparing the AIDS situation to the cholera epidemic in Toronto in 1832—he had been coached on this subject by his friend Bert Hansen, who taught at U of T's Institute for the History and Philosophy of Science and Technology. Moral judgements on lifestyle were popular at the time of the cholera epidemic, and immigrants were blamed for the outbreak. The cause was held to be dirt, and whole ships of immigrants were quarantined. Lynch compared the reactions to cholera to the "hubbub back in February over so-called 'gay blood' bans."

In the case of AIDS, he continued:

> We have seen equivalent prejudices. The early labelling of AIDS as a "gay plague" persists today. The myth that gays are the villains, infecting the pure "general population" also continues, suppressing the appalling central fact: that we are the main sufferers of a horrendous disease. . . . With revolutionary openness we have

fought a homophobic society that wanted us back in our closets. Ahead of us now are major tasks of standing up to a society which seeks to make us passive victims by scaring us and fostering panic among us.

Lynch observed that in the months since his November 1982 article in *The Body Politic*, "a great deal of community mobilization and debate" had occurred. The mandate was now clear. The community had eight ways of responding: keep informed; make careful choices in health-care matters; challenge anti-gay biases; pressure public health agencies and governments; support AIDS patients; help people who had a fear of getting AIDS; make sure there were gay participants in public health forums; and do fundraising.

Lynch especially stressed the need to challenge homophobia. "More sex, better sex, *safe* sex should be one of our goals. When our sexual lives are under siege is when we most need to be out of the closet about this goal." At the same time, AIDS patients needed support: counselling, transportation, housework, and a guarantee of their rights in hospitals. Lynch concluded: "A basic choice confronts us: scared, we can run off to hide in the shadows and cower, or we can organize to bring our fight for gay health, for active gay sexuality, and for gay love and gay pride into the public eye."

"Good to see you back on the platform," Ed Jackson told Lynch after the meeting. "After your retirement."

In his speech, despite his antagonism towards Hamburg's views, Lynch made his first ever written reference to "safe sex" (although without mentioning condoms). A diary entry explains why: his speech was *"a lecture to say what a committee thought I should say. It was right to say it so, strategically sound . . ."* Apparently, after the speech was delivered his efforts evoked praise for being so *"rational"* and *"middle of the road."*

After the three main speakers, the Jarvis meeting broke down into smaller groups to discuss issues related to committee work. At one of these smaller groups, Peter Evans identified himself as someone with AIDS. Evans, twenty-eight, hailed from Ottawa but had been working in England as a stage designer. In December 1982 he had become the first person in England diagnosed as having AIDS.[5]

A seven-point AIDS strategy: Toronto's Public Health Department

Bill Mindell and Dr. Richard Fralick of the City of Toronto's Public Health Department attended the packed Jarvis meeting. "What an eye opener. People were along the aisles and in the back," Mindell said. The next day Mindell was the spokesperson as Toronto's Public Health Department held a press conference to announce its seven-point strategy for AIDS, the first such strategy of its kind in Canada.[6] Modelled after an approach developed in San Francisco and devised in co-operation with U of T AIDS researchers, the strategy was spearheaded by a public health team headed by Mindell, co-ordinator of community health information for the department, along with Fralick, associate medical officer of health, and public relations co-ordinator Anne Moon.

The first item in the strategy was to develop, in collaboration with Hassle Free Clinic, a pamphlet and poster campaign to inform the gay community of risks and symptoms of AIDS. Part of this was the "Numbers" campaign, which urged gay men to reduce the number of their sexual partners and featured a poster with men at a bar in silhouette. The other points included informing health department staff how to advise the public on AIDS, reassuring laboratory staff about standard protective procedures, liaising with other government committees, and reassuring the public about the small risk of getting AIDS.[7] Peter Evans agreed to participate in the press conference, although he did not reveal his last name. *The Globe and Mail* did a separate story about him to accompany the press conference report. "Peter, six feet three inches tall, fair haired, with a gentle, vulnerable face, is 28 years old, but looks younger," the *Globe and Mail* article stated, before detailing Evans's experience with AIDS.[8]

When Mindell joined the department in 1983, public health had stopped focusing on infectious diseases, including sexually transmitted diseases, and was instead increasingly concerning itself with "lifestyle" diseases resulting from tobacco use, the polluted environment, and other factors, he said. "The idea was that communicable diseases were history." Despite the high number of STDs in the gay community, in the long run, they thought, "it was a small community and STDs were hundreds of years old." The department was bent on taking a new approach to public health. As a result, AIDS "was not in the business plan, so it was a crisis kind of response," he said. As the latest recruit to the department, Mindell had the least on his plate, and he took over the AIDS portfolio. He also had a personal interest in the syndrome. His son had recently been diagnosed as having hemophilia. Meanwhile, the province's chief medical officer of health, David Korn, remained silent on the subject of AIDS, and there was a conscious effort to keep the issue, associated as it was with gays and sex, away from Health Minister Larry Grossman.

"The gay community clearly took the leadership in the early days," Mindell said. Within public health, Mindell, Fralick, and Moon were active. "But we weren't the chiefs, and no money was flowing," he said. "If this had been considered important, money would have flowed." By August Mindell had dubbed AIDS an "emerging epidemic" in the city.[9]

With his teaching over for the school year, Lynch had once again made plans for the summer. This time he wouldn't be going away. In addition to settling into his new house, where work was behind schedule and costs were escalating, he wanted to read the multi-volume *Remembrance of Things Past* by Marcel Proust and play the piano. He needed a break from AIDS, he wrote in his diary in July. *"All I want to do is practice Mozart."* But July was a busy month. It began with a disco fundraiser for the new AIDS committee held at Stages and included, for Lynch, a health scare. Early in the month he woke up wanting to die, *"aching with sleeplessness and the enchainement of fatigue."* He had a tightness in his chest— *"a contraction in breathing and in the self . . . A hot lemony sugary infusion calms me, but lungs are baby lungs."* He wondered if he might be showing signs of PCP.

His sale of Roehampton and temporary move to the Riverdale house, and all the rest of the activity, had left him without a lot of time to deal with the deaths of his mother and grandmother. *"Oh, to clear the agenda for a direct management of fatigue, despair—and grief. The grief won't go away. I have been friable,"* he wrote. He found himself breaking into tears over his mother and grandmother as well as the long-ago loss of Base (his Aunt Mabel). *"The great blank, in Stevens, the basic slate, even Anangke. Why? Why 'go on'?"*[10] A few days later, after a dream about visiting his mother and Base in a *"terminal hospital,"* he mused, *"As you get older, does all experience become a network of dying?"*

The AIDS Committee makes its debut

On July 12 Lynch was elected to the executive of the AIDS Committee of Toronto. Also elected were his "preferred candidates"—Bert Hansen, Bill Lewis, Stephen Fontaine, and Robert Trow. *"Bill earlier asked if I would be chair—that scares me. Is my typewriter-activist period ended? I'm scared that it, like the Damien committee, could rob me from myself."* Two days later Lynch probably heaved a sigh of relief when Hansen was elected as the first chair of the AIDS Committee.

The AIDS Committee of Toronto made its formal debut at a press conference on July 19. The event was designed, among other things, to "let people know that there was now an organized response to AIDS . . . and some coordination and communication amongst the various players at the time," Ed Jackson told the Krever Commission.[11] But Peter Evans, the Ottawa theatre designer who had AIDS, captured much of the media attention. Handsome and articulate, the young man had become the first person in Canada to speak publicly about his condition. "'Peter,' from Ottawa, is the first person the media wants to talk to at the press conference," reported *NOW*, a Toronto weekly newsmagazine. "A man in his late twenties, he faces the banks of television cameras."[12] Cecchi was also front and centre at the press conference, as were ACT members Hansen, Robert Wallace, and Karsten Kossmann. Bill Mindell of Toronto's Public Health Department was also there, along with other notables: Dr. Roslyn Herst of the Canadian Red Cross Society; and doctors Colin Soskolne, Stan Read, and Randy Coates of the University of Toronto AIDS Research team.

ACT very clearly emerged from Toronto's gay community, but the press conference organizers, true to their appointed mandate, were careful to alert other affected groups—Haitian organizations, the Canadian Hemophilia Society—and invite them to attend the event. Organizers were also careful to supply background information and direction to the media. A media kit for the press conference, prepared in large part by Lynch, included a number of inserts: a copy of the so-called "Denver Principles" (Statement from People with AIDS); a chronology of AIDS in Canada (authored by Lynch); and some pointers for journalists writing about AIDS. The notes for journalists reminded them, for example, that AIDS was occurring in a number of populations and that phrases such as "gay plague" or "gay epidemic," even in quotes, were therefore "inaccurate and misleading." The kit also contained an annotated copy of an article from the journal *Nature*, and an updated list of AIDS figures.

Having Roslyn Herst at the press conference was like an endorsement, a kind of Good Housekeeping seal of approval for the new organization. But Herst didn't follow the expected script. She was a last-minute substitute for John Derrick of the Red Cross Society, and briefed herself using a confidential background Q and A sheet that the Public Health Department had prepared. One answer in that sheet stated, for instance, that "until more is known, individuals belonging to groups at higher than normal risk of developing A.I.D.S. are asked to refrain from donating blood."[13]

The next day *The Toronto Sun* story began not with the story of Peter Evans, or the announcement of the new organization, but with remarks from Herst. The newspaper reported that, according to Herst, "It is now 'unofficial policy' to discourage homosexuals from donating blood until AIDS-causing agents can be identified and procedures to test for the agents in blood can be developed." *NOW* newsmagazine elaborated on the same matter, quoting Herst as saying that the request for all gay men to refrain from donating was not the official policy of the Red Cross, but that since so much was unknown about the disease, "It would be prudent for homosexual men, whether monogamous, celibate or whatever, not to donate blood."[14]

Activists were furious with this statement, which seemed to reflect an apparent change in policy. They had fought hard to have the Red Cross articulate a policy stating that not all homosexuals— but only sexually active homosexuals with multiple partners—refrain from donating blood. An emergency meeting with ACT and the Red Cross was called for the next day.

On the same day as the ACT press conference, the Ontario Ministry of Health announced a $500,000 fund for research on AIDS, with $100,000 of it already allocated to a University of Toronto study proposed by a team including doctors Coates and Soskolne. The study would follow the symptom-free sexual partners of gay men diagnosed as having either AIDS or an AIDS-related complex (ARC).

The emergency meeting with the Red Cross, attended by Hansen, Lynch, Mindell, and Derrick, dissolved into acrimony. Hansen became angry at Derrick's apparent failure to understand the issue of the possible stigmatization of gay community. "My concern was that if they could blame a disease on us, we were in trouble as a community. So that is why we were so outraged by the Red Cross for not accepting gay and lesbian blood. We said you're smearing us all, that kind of headline encourages gay bashers and other kinds of homophobes." Jackson later speculated that Hansen's outburst at the meeting "probably coloured the Red Cross's interpretation of how touchy the gay community was from that point on."[15] Just a half-year or so later, Derrick would note: "As you are aware, our experience w/reference to inviting representatives of high-risk groups to meet . . . has been *extremely difficult* and not very fruitful . . . the disruptive effects of non-scientific issues have been extensive."

After the meeting with the Red Cross, at a hastily convened press conference on the steps of the Ontario legislature, Lynch set out to clarify the "erroneous and distorted" media reports on the Red Cross policy on blood donations and to ridicule the provincial funding announcement. "The Red Cross informed us that its blood-donor policy set last March 10 has not changed," the July 20 release stated. "AIDS has no inherent relation to sexual orientation, and sexual orientation has no inherent connection with any disease." Lynch told the press that the budget for the U of T AIDS study was $1.7 million and the announcement of $100,000 funding from the province was a "laughable, hollow gesture." He argued that Keith Norton, who had replaced Larry Grossman as Ontario's health minister in early July, was trying to distract the public from "the real issue: his refusal to take seriously the need for AIDS funding in Ontario."

That evening Lynch told his diary: "*AIDS all day. Flurry over press in A.M. Meeting, emergency, with Red Cross in p.m. Then over gin lemon-*

ades at Bert's, he Bill and I put together a press release. Several phone interviews, but basically they [media] *all met me at steps . . . I'm falling asleep. National TV (CTV) tomorrow A.M. Must be up at 6:30."*

Although Lynch and ACT blamed the media for reporting "errors," they had been upset about Herst's actual remarks. The July 26 minutes of ACT's executive committee, for example, described Herst's comments at the press conference as "unacceptable, discriminatory and socially dangerous." According to Dale McCarthy, at the time vice-chair of ACT, other members of the executive committee were not as upset as Lynch, Lewis, and Hansen about Herst's remarks. The committee had gone through a lively discussion, McCarthy said, "about the fine distinction between all homosexuals on one side, and promiscuous homosexuals or homosexuals with multiple partners on the other," as well as talking about the importance of "all that differentiating."[16] (A couple of months earlier, Mindell had unsuccessfully urged the Red Cross to ask for the voluntary exclusion of all gay and bisexual men from donating blood. He argued that the proviso that only the sexually active be asked to exclude themselves "weakens and confuses" the policy.[17] It was already known, and had been reported by Lewis in *The Body Politic*, that some men who developed AIDS had very few partners, and also that there was a carrier state.) For its part, the Canadian Red Cross Society issued its own press release on July 22, essentially disavowing Herst's statements and confirming that only "sexually-active homosexual or bisexual men with multiple partners need refrain from donating blood."[18]

A convergence of activities

At the beginning of August ACT hired two more staff, Gary Kinsman and Sarah Yates-Howorth, and moved to offices at 66 Wellesley Street East, above a Kentucky Fried Chicken outlet.

Lynch stayed in Toronto most of the rest of the summer, occasionally attending ACT meetings and speaking to the media about AIDS. He was also settling into his new home on Ross Street. His apartment occupied the entire ground floor and the front two-thirds of the second floor area of the house, with Lewis's apartment taking up the balance of the second floor and the third floor. Lynch's ground floor was designed to showcase his grand piano, which was situated near the base of a freestanding metal staircase that ascended to Lynch's bedroom perch at the front of the house. (The "bedroom" was an open area.) His study area wrapped around part of the second floor's side wall, leaving a two-storey ceiling height for most of the open-concept apartment.[19] Stefan's main-floor bedroom allowed for privacy—it had walls and a door. It also opened onto the back garden.

Lynch continued to read *Remembrance of Things Past* through the summer. In his July 29 diary entry, he transcribed a passage from volume II:

> . . . *death is not in vain.* . . . *The dead continue to act upon us. They act upon us even more than the living because, true reality being discoverable only by the mind ... we acquire a true knowledge only of things that we are obliged to recreate by thought, things that are hidden from us in everyday life.*

Stefan, now eleven, returned from his summer in California near the end of August, having grown so much since he left Toronto that, at the airport, his father didn't immediately recognize him, at first mistaking him for a teenage girl—*"in a bobbed haircut and boyish trousers and sports jacket."* (By the time he reached his grown height of six feet, two inches tall, Stefan towered over his five-foot-eight father.) Lynch recorded the odd sensation of thinking, as Stefan walked through the long airport corridor, *"that he, my son, is my father."* That evening he explored that moment in his diary: *"Stefan is my father because no one else in the whole world whom I know has my genes, my interior sculptors, in Proust's metaphor, and I look to him to see what I reflect in my own fiz and manners, as a house might look to its plans, or another house from similar plans: the order of building isn't crucial."*

During the day that summer Lynch taught part-time at Erindale, grateful to pick up extra English classes to help pay for renovations. A professor by day, Lynch got back into his nocturnal disco-going habit and mused on his opposing instincts towards solitude—*"I drift toward it only, not make an active choice"*—and an active sexual life: *"I nearly feel that it is illicit—not admissible—**not** to be tricking, **not** to have sex several times a week with someone."* A few days later, feeling drained of energy, he considered the possibility that he had AIDS and saw a certain irony in his new "showpiece" house, which he had several times jokingly called his "coffin."

Just a day or two earlier, he said, he had remarked to someone that it had been two years since he had probably been exposed to AIDS—a full two years since he had last stayed at The Pines on Fire Island. *"I hope I can think I've self-immunized,"* he wrote. So little was then known about AIDS that it seemed a reasonable theory that whatever caused AIDS was like a regular virus, and a person could build up antibodies and become immune. Still, he wondered to himself how he would spend his time if he got sick. *"Quit teaching? Work full-time on the novel? . . . My needs re Stefan, re friends. Stefan I postpone thinking about."* He wondered if he would keep it to himself until a diagnosis was firm: *"(Or would I? I'd wanna tell Bill). Bill would be the most important of all, and I'd really need/want him to be actively involved in my illness and (for this may safely be presumed) dying."* He also pondered suicide—*"The only problem is **where** . . . I'd prefer home, here, in this bed . . ."* He would prepare his friends, too: for *"living after me: for 'closure,' for not dying with me, for a newer sense of the vitality of living after I'm dead, for remembering me in an enlivening, not a mortifying, way."*

Lynch acknowledged that AIDS had not (yet) led him to behave any differently, not made him any "pickier" as he left bars. He still had about the same amount of sex and number of partners as in the summer of 1981 at Fire Island. He still found that *"the aggressive loneliness (didn't I call it so then?) persists in the self, though the understanding of it changes."*

In early fall, when he resumed his full teaching load, Lynch continued going out to discos and clubs and doing recreational drugs. In early October came a convergence of his activities: *"Gentling down today from the MDA I've been up, giggly, dancing naked in front of the bathroom mirror to 'I Will Survive' before my shower, enjoying the new toy as I (for the first time) word processed terminal remarks to essays I was reading (lost 2 remarks, thanks to disk overload)."* These were still early days for home computers, and Lynch had bought one at the urging of Stefan, who from an early age was the computer expert in the family.

Hansen resigned as chair of ACT on September 27, just over two months after he was elected. A month earlier, Lynch attended an emergency meeting of ACT, a meeting necessitated (he told his diary) by Hansen's extraordinary thoroughness: *"Bert's mind sees everything in a mega-powerful spotlight and his will wants everything to be chosen with full consciousness. No sliding, no shadows, no sloppiness."* Hansen told the committee he was resigning because fundamental problems were being ignored or denied. ACT needed firmer priorities. "My worries are primarily about structure and planning and making decisions, yet these problems have been perceived as personal rather than systemic." As a result, he said, he would remove himself from the executive and make comments "from the safety of the sidelines."[20] Years later Hansen said a major concern for him was a lack of clarity about the respective roles of the board of directors and the staff. In the wake of Hansen's resignation, Dr. Dale McCarthy became interim chair.

Meanwhile, the Toronto Public Health Department continued to develop policy about the emerging epidemic. In an August 1983 document—"not intended to be publicly distributed or regarded as policy positions of the Department of Health"—the department articulated a number of important positions.[21] The San Francisco public health department was being pressured to close bathhouses or bars in order to curb the spread of AIDS, but Toronto rejected that approach. According to the document, such places were not in themselves responsible for the spread of AIDS and the very fact of their existence gave the department "an obvious place to distribute our literature and put up the posters that can inform the gay male community of the risks involved. Without such gathering places, it would be harder to keep the community informed."[22] A long-standing precedent existed for this practice; Hassle Free Clinic had done STD prevention work in the city's bars and bathhouses for years.

ACT's attempt to include representatives of other "high-risk" groups in the organization proved far from easy. Dale Moauro, a man with hemophilia, attended ACT meetings as an observer, but he was not an official representative of the Canadian Hemophilia Society. Indeed, ACT was told that the Ontario and Metro chapters of the Society were operating under a "gag order" from the national executive.

They had been told that only the national organization could speak about AIDS-related issues.[23] Nevertheless, ACT passed a motion that a representative of the hemophiliac community be invited to sit on the executive, and that other members of that community be invited to join working groups. ACT also made overtures to members of the Haitian community in Toronto.

ACT received its letters patent on October 4, and on the same day its charitable status became effective. The applicants were listed as Bert Hansen, Stephen Fontaine, Bill Lewis, Robert Trow, and Michael Lynch. Nine days later Bert Hansen addressed a public health seminar on AIDS at the invitation of Toronto's medical officer of health, Sandy Macpherson. Hansen took the opportunity to applaud the work of the department. "As an historian, I want to observe first that in the three years of AIDS through the United States, public health workers, especially at the municipal level, have consistently had the quickest and most sane responses to problems. . . . Toronto fits that same pattern, and for this I am most grateful." But he went on to stress the need to "normalize" AIDS as a disease, and to counter those who would use it to reinforce prejudices—people who refer to the disease as "divine judgement," for example. "With AIDS I find that professionals often prefer to ignore these unscientific and vicious claims in the pulpit, the press, and on TV," Hansen said. "No matter how silly they are, ideas not challenged will not just go away. My point here is that such claims must be challenged, not only by the groups that are slandered, but by the professionals."[24]

At ACT's second general meeting on October 18 the city's Public Health Department presented its AIDS poster and pamphlet campaign—the "Numbers" campaign—that it had developed with the participation of the Hassle Free Clinic, as previewed at ACT's July press conference. Lynch told the assembled group, "We have to dig in our heels for the long haul." They needed, he said, to learn to work with government, the media, the Hemophilia Society, and the Haitian community.

Less than two weeks later, Lynch acted on that commitment. At an October 27 meeting with Ministry of Health officials, he turned the floor over to Bill Mindell, who on that occasion was representing the Canadian Hemophilia Society. Mindell made the case for the development of a comprehensive care plan for hemophiliacs, since it was becoming clear that they would be hard hit by AIDS.[25]

Take 30, a CBC-Toronto current affairs TV program, was one of the first to air Canadian programs about AIDS. In March 1983 it ran a medically oriented program featuring Read and Derrick. A program the following November examined the impact of AIDS on individuals and communities. Cecchi, Lynch, Moauro, and Hamburg appeared on the program, although they were not identified by name. Lynch told of an intelligent woman friend who had asked him if it was safe to rent out her apartment to anyone else, since the previous tenant had had AIDS.

By late 1983 the issue of safe sex had moved firmly front and centre. In "Is There Safe Sex?", a major article in *The Body Politic's* final issue of the year, writer Rick Bébout outlined the logic behind the advice to use condoms for anal sex—although he quoted a doctor who pointed out that the efficacy of condoms had not yet been proven. In the article Bébout surveyed the science and interviewed doctors and gay activists, providing a snapshot of the late 1983 state of knowledge. After outlining the most up-to-date advice being given, he then questioned it. To advise people to "limit the number of different sexual partners" was a matter of simple logic, he noted, if you accepted the single-agent theory of AIDS. But that advice didn't tell anyone *what* to do with the people they have sex with. The rule of choosing a sexual partner carefully, he pointed out, did not tell you on what basis you should make this choice.[26] ACT decided Bébout's article was so important that the organization ordered extra copies to send to people on its mailing list.

Around this time ACT published a one-page advice sheet, "Condoms: Gay men try them on for size," which provided advice about shopping for condoms: "The first thing to remember is that you're a gay man, these things weren't made for you, and you're using someone else's toys. Don't avoid a package just because it looks more heterosexual." It also reported the reactions of various "testers," most of whom were trying condoms for the first time—some objected to the smell of latex condoms, some found lubrication insufficient—and suggested practising their use: "Wear a rubber next time you are jacking off . . . eventually, the rubber won't bother you . . . so keep trying, just don't expect instant perfection."

During this busy period Stefan was having a difficult time. One evening, after a mishap when he tried to move a television by himself, he broke down in a *"long aching painful cry,"* insisting he was nothing but a pest and everyone would be better off if he ran away to the Yukon. Lynch reassured his eleven-year-old, telling him how much he wanted him to be with him. After telling him of the anguish of his own childhood, he noted, *"I spoke of my conviction in periods of deep depression that nothing would change. I told him, eye to eye, that I love him far more than out of paternal obligation."*

As 1983 drew to a close, Lynch remarked to Ed Jackson that he hadn't written a thing in a year. "You can't write and be a party girl," Jackson replied.[27]

When he was heading to New York to spend Christmas there, Lynch realized that Toronto was beginning to feel like home. Writing about himself in the third person, he asked: *"Did he not, now, with 8 Ross Street under his head, did he not feel like Toronto was reaching in and taking hold? Was he giving up his citizenship in his home country— not legally, now, but in his heart—to become a citizen of Ross St., a small domestic enclave in a medium sized city north of the lake?"* But by the time he had spent a couple of days in New York he was writing: *"No doubt about it, this is home. I must plan, plan, plan to get here on or before retirement."*

Stefan had gone to California, to spend Christmas with his mother and Pat Bond. After Bond and Lynch had chatted on the telephone for a while, she asked, *"Do you want to speak to your family?"* *"I am talking to my family,"* he replied.

Lynch spent Christmas day with Spiers and his partner Ray Gray. Spiers had a second-floor loft, and Gray an eighth-floor studio apartment in the same building on 19th Street in New York. A storage elevator connected the two lofts. *"Herb summoned me to Ray's, whose table lacked no presents for the three of us,"* Lynch wrote. Later Gray, who wasn't feeling well, stayed home while Spiers and Lynch headed off to have Christmas dinner with friends Bruce Schentes and David Cohen. The two hosts *"proved how well two Jews, if schooled by all the proper homo boys, could throw a yuletide better than the goys."* It was during the holidays that Lynch made plans to spend an upcoming sabbatical year (1984–85) in New York. But before that, he would have to stickhandle through various crises at the AIDS Committee of Toronto.

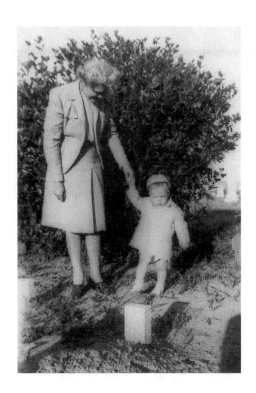

Toddler Mike Lynch (he became "Michael" when he went to college) and Mabel ("Base"), his favourite aunt, at a gravestone. Mabel and her companion, Esther, taught Michael to cook and garden (courtesy of CLGA archives).

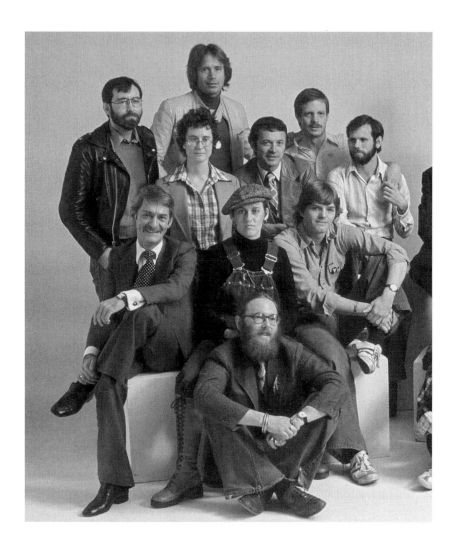

Another photo from this session was published as a centrespread in the Dec. 17, 1977, issue of Weekend Magazine *with the caption "Gay in the Seventies." It accompanied an article, with the same title, by Ian Young. The individuals in the photo were identified as:*

BACK ROW: Ian Young, author, Toronto; Trevor Montford Smith, engineer, Ontario Hydro, Toronto; John Alan Lee, author and sociologist, University of Toronto; Michael Lynch, assistant professor, University of Toronto; Bill Lewis, microbiologist, University of Toronto; Edgar Z. Friedenberg, author and professor, Dalhousie University, Halifax; Jim Quixley, head librarian, Glendon College, York University, Toronto; David Gibson, graphic artist and civil servant, Toronto; David Garmaise, division manager of Canada Post, Ottawa; Clarence Barnes, chemical engineer, University of Toronto.

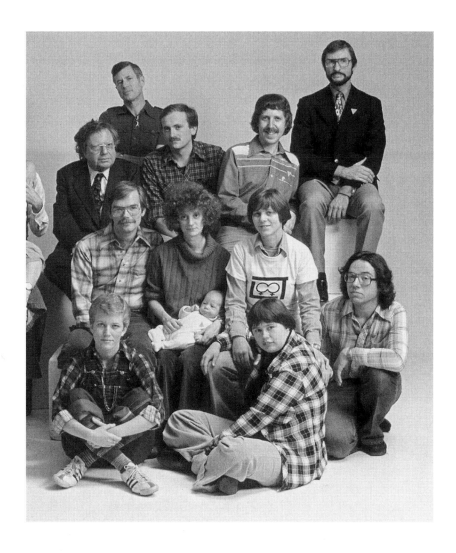

Middle row: Ron Shearer, businessman, Toronto; Dr. Rosemary Barnes, psychologist, Toronto General Hospital; Marie Robertson, federal civil servant, Ottawa; Mark Whitehead, university student, Toronto; Ed Jackson, researcher, Ontario Institute for Studies in Education, Toronto; Theresa Faubert (with her baby Jodie), teacher, Toronto; Konnie Reich, photo lab technician, Toronto; Stuart Russell, typesetter, Montreal.

Front row: Charles Hill, assistant curator, National Gallery, Ottawa; Debbie Parent, clerk, Bell Canada, Ottawa; Christine Bearchell, office worker, Toronto.

(Photo: Croydon/Reeves)

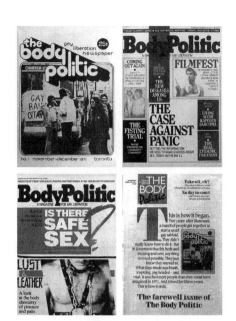

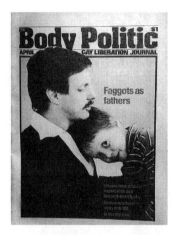

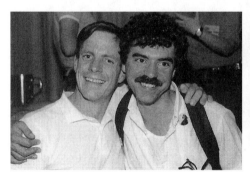

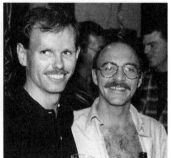

Top LEFT: *Body Politic* covers courtesy of Pink Triangle Press

Top RIGHT: *Michael Lynch and his six-year-old son, Stefan. Lynch's feature article "Forgotten Fathers," in this 1978 issue of* The Body Politic, *led to the formation of Gay Fathers Toronto* (courtesy of Pink Triangle Press).

BOTTOM LEFT: *Michael Lynch and historian Allan Bérubé at the Wilde '82 ("Doing It") conference in Toronto. It was the first international gathering of gay and lesbian historians* (courtesy of Pink Triangle Press).

BOTTOM RIGHT: *Microbiologist Bill Lewis and epidemiologist and doctor Randy Coates relaxing at a party, probably in the early 1980s. Both men were involved in early AIDS research, and both died from AIDS-related causes* (courtesy of Pink Triangle Press).

four

SWANSONG TO ACTIVISM?

*I see my generation marching, or **demonstrating**, its way down Yonge Street, with a sound track & with posters & placards & cheering and printed balloons, towards the country of the dead. Hades, yesterday a name with a quaint mythy scent to it, like an old dress from the attic closet, today is a region beginning just at the end of the street, where I know many inhabitants.*
— Michael Lynch, Diary no. 39, November 1, 1983

Peter Evans, the young man *The Body Politic* had dubbed Canada's "National Person with AIDS," died on January 7, 1984, only six months after he went public about having AIDS. At the time Evans was the thirty-fifth Canadian known to have died of AIDS. Even as his health was suffering, Evans had continued to "put a face on AIDS." He appeared at press conferences in Winnipeg, Toronto, and Ottawa, gave scores of media interviews, and spoke at many public forums. It was important for Evans to speak out about AIDS "from an emotional standpoint," said his Ottawa doctor, John Henderson. "He felt obliged to communicate the thoughts and feelings of somebody who did have this problem, in the hope that it might be helpful to fellow sufferers."[1]

Despite his expressed fears about doing so, Lynch had just assumed a six-month term as chair of the ACT board, and his first official task was to represent the organization at Evans's funeral. The night before he flew to Ottawa, Lynch wrote in his diary: *"Burying people gets less & less special. In middle age, one becomes a part-time pallbearer."*

After attending the service at the funeral home (named, *"with a Waughish humour,"* Fairplay), Lynch dutifully went back to the family home. *"I felt like a lawyer, especially with my dark suit and shoes,"* he wrote, *"while they, by this point, were in at-home mufti."* The family promised to give the funeral donations to ACT. *"I had gone to offer fellow-feeling, and felt a bit like I had come to pick up the stash,"* Lynch said. Despite the painful experience the family had been through— as horrible as Larry Okin's death, Lynch thought—there was only min- imal talk of AIDS, or of Peter. It was as though Peter had *"just left for a month in London."* Mrs. Evans showed Lynch two wooden Easter eggs Peter had painted, Ukrainian-style, for her, and *"wondered rather casually"* where her son had left other bits of his artwork. *"In the basement? In the box in the bedroom? In England, with X, his lover?"* Peter's aunt, his mother's sister, *"sat bolt upright w/legs bent, knees together, on the sofa by the fire, knitting."* She thought she had some of Peter's batik or block prints, but had never before seen the eggs. *"Mr. Evans' back has a problem, but still he splits wood and heats—except for this year with sick Peter there—the suburban Ottawa middle class house, with a wood furnace in the basement. He put on several good size logs of elm that he'd split."* The conversation turned to heating methods, and to the Victorian house in the country belonging to Roddie (Peter's gay brother), who apparently had rather *"kooky decorating ideas (barn- wood wainscotting in the kitchen?)."* They talked about people who didn't show up at the funeral home.

For the rest of his life, Lynch would be visiting hospitals, sitting at deathbeds, and regularly attending funerals and memorial ser- vices. His visit with the Evans would stand out, though, because it was on the family's turf. Usually when Lynch met the parents of friends who had died, it was on neutral ground, not at family homes. So many friends had, like himself, emigrated from smaller centres to Toronto, New York, and San Francisco, leaving parents and extended family behind in a bid to find, as gay men, a level of comfort and community. Sometimes, as well, families were not accepting of their sons' sexual orientation. Evans, as a gay man, had been fully accepted and loved by his parents.

Just two days after Lynch returned from Ottawa, Robert Gildenhuys, a former lover, telephoned. He sounded down, and there was a long, unaccustomed silence after their initial greeting. Lynch was "slow to twig" to what was going on. Then it came out. Gildenhuys said a Chicago friend of his had just called to say he had AIDS.

Crises at ACT: money and "the dark of bureaucracy"

The media sensationalism and fear about AIDS that had character-ized 1983 died down somewhat in 1984, even as AIDS cases contin-ued to increase steadily. On November 25, 1983, Health Canada's Laboratory Centre for Disease Control (LCDC) had received reports of 51 AIDS cases in the country. In a November 2, 1984 update, the LCDC reported 147 cases. Early in the year, CBC-Television's *National News* aired a five-part series of "Special Reports," three to four minutes long, on AIDS. ACT staff had spent a lot of time responding to media queries and helped the CBC team with research, but noticeably absent from the series was any mention of Toronto gay community involve-ment and organizing around AIDS. ACT decided, in March, to protest this omission. The series "implied there is little awareness of and/or reaction to the crisis by Metro's gay men. The opposite is true—as is signified by the existence of our organization," ACT wrote in a letter to the CBC. "We are shocked that you should ignore the work and commitment of a volunteer organization that to a large degree sup-plied the information that made your program possible."[2]

ACT continued to benefit from an alliance with Bill Mindell and his team in Toronto's Department of Public Health, and the organi-zation was also developing better relations with the province. One of the first things that Keith Norton did after he became Ontario health minister in the summer of 1983 was to visit U.S. AIDS researchers at the Centers for Disease Control in Atlanta and the National Institutes for Health near Washington, D.C.[3] Norton was a closeted gay man (he came out publicly years later). His executive assistant, Doug Bonnell, also a gay man, became an insider ally to the cause of AIDS and would go on to become chair of the board of the AIDS Committee of Toronto in 1989.

But ACT faced both internal and external crises in the first half of 1984. The internal crisis developed out of differences about how the organization should operate. Key players in the group's formation had previously been associated with organizations that worked as collectives—*The Body Politic*, Hassle Free Clinic, and the Right to Privacy Committee. Yet from the beginning, thanks to the federal job employment grant, ACT had employees. At first, in keeping with a collective model, they had no titles, recalled Karsten Kossmann. "But we were dealing with a big epidemic. We would need government funds and alliances with other organizations . . . so for that purpose, when we contacted the world out there, when we wrote letters, we needed to at least have titles." The initial employees—Kossmann, who had previously worked as an executive secretary, freelance writer Sarah Yates-Howorth, and gay activist and academic Gary Kinsman— had identical salaries and were soon given titles: office manager, media officer, and education officer. But they were told to continue operating as a collective.

Yates-Howorth was soon put in charge of liaison among staff, volunteers, and the board. When she asked for a pay raise in recognition of those extra responsibilities she was harshly criticized by several board members, and some staffing committee members who supported her walked out of an early February meeting in protest. Yates-Howorth quit. Lynch had been one of her critics. He had, for one thing, objected to her writing style. He wanted her to write academically, not journalistically. He recognized, though, that in league with Bill Lewis and Bert Hansen he tended to be a "staff basher," and that the staff would need an advocate committee to shield them from the bashing. Lynch realized that he "mercilessly" wounded Sarah's pride and self-respect. Clearly disturbed by his own behaviour, he saw himself *"as prideful and arrogant and comfortable and disdainful of others and untrusting and manipulating and untrustworthy."*

A few days after Yates-Howorth gave notice, Lynch met with her in a bid to have her stay on. She refused, but continued to work with ACT as a volunteer. Kossmann said her gender and sexual orientation might have also been a strike against her. Best friends with Randy Coates, Yates-Howorth was comfortable with gay men, but some board members questioned the appropriateness of ACT being represented by a heterosexual woman. This point became moot when Joan Anderson, a heterosexual, went on to become chair of the board and later a key staff member at ACT. Lesbians were also central to the organization in its early days. Psychologist Rosemary Barnes was a key figure in AIDS Support, the caregiving wing of ACT, and so too were Theresa Dobko and Yvette Perreault.

All the turmoil in the organization took its toll. *"ACT has gone into the dark of bureaucracy and I am its undertaker, civil servant,"* Lynch told his diary. By that point Bill Lewis was threatening to resign. *"Bill can't work with people so different from himself in their assumptions. I who call this my swansong to activism—wish I had steered clear of all of this."* Lewis did quit the board in March, citing time restrictions.

Meanwhile, ACT was facing a funding crisis and Lynch and others were trying hard to find money for the organization. In mid-March ACT applied for $180,000 from the federal government (the grant was refused), and Lynch sent a letter accompanied by a review of ACT's work over the previous eight months. Next he wrote seeking funding to Health Minister Norton in early April. The letter began, "Dear Keith, I'm looking ahead to the end of the tunnel and trying to find the door. . . . If there is no door at the end of the tunnel, it seems, the entire system will suffer. Who will take distress calls? Correct media misinformation? Provide speakers to a wide range of groups? Counsel and/or refer those with AIDS and those with fear of AIDS?"[4] Meanwhile, ACT had found an ally in another Progressive Conservative, Susan Fish, the provincial minister of citizenship and culture and MPP for St. George, the downtown Toronto riding where ACT was located.

Death and night sweats

On Tuesday, March 13, 1984, Lynch slept in, puttered about the house, and then in a late afternoon snowfall walked east to Yonge Street with Stephen, a young disc jockey who had spent the night with him. The two of them had recently begun a relationship. After Stephen went off home, Lynch continued on to ACT's office on Wellesley Street, just west of Church Street. When ACT moved to that location the landlord asked that the group limit any signage to a small window display—which was not a problem because ACT did not want to advertise its presence. It wanted to protect the privacy of visitors and keep a low profile. When the organization first occupied the premises it had received bomb and fire threats.

At ACT Lynch took care of *"letters and interviews and hiring and more letters"* when what he really wanted to do was go to the gym and work out. The snow had stopped falling by the time he walked home, and just as he stepped in the door the phone was ringing. It was Herb Spiers calling, and Lynch asked him to hold while he got out of his snowy shoes. *"You don't sound good,"* Lynch said. His first thought was that Herb was "reacting badly" to the plan being pursued for his upcoming sabbatical in New York: Lynch was going to stay in Herb's apartment. But then Spiers told Lynch about Herb's lover Ray Gray. Ray was in Mount Sinai Hospital, diagnosed with PCP, perhaps with AIDS. While they were still on the phone Ray's parents called Spiers. *"Herb had to break off and lie to them, only half successfully,"* Lynch wrote. When Lynch rang back Spiers *"spoke of cracked plastic seats in a slow emergency waiting room, of IV tubes & oxygen masks."* Apparently he had called Lynch the evening before, but Lynch had somehow missed hearing the message.

Five days later, on March 18, Bill Lewis had his thirty-fourth birthday. Lynch, Michael Pearl, Greg Bourgeois, Yves Dufour, and Gerald Hannon celebrated it over brunch at Fenton's, one of Toronto's fanciest restaurants, complete with a birthday cake for dessert. When he arrived back home, Lynch had phone messages telling him that Gray was much worse. Within an hour, he was in a limo on his way to the airport. Once there he managed to get on a standby flight to New York.

After a long session at the hospital with Gray on March 20, Spiers and Lynch went to Central Park and walked around the reservoir. It was clear that Gray was dying. They talked about Ray Gray and his many moods: *"campy, designing, lazing, playing."* Gray's imminent death, Spiers thought, was bound to bring about estate problems. His father Jack Gray was an ex-cop, *"real hot to trot."* They talked about Herb and his memories, his prospects. Spiers mentioned

Bruce Schentes's quick move to David Cohen after Larry Okin died, and his own doubts that he could love or be loved by anyone again. They went for a beer and Spiers asked Lynch what he should say to Ray—he might only get a few more chances to talk to him—and Lynch asked him what he would want to hear from Ray if it were him on his deathbed. *"He got into that."*

Lynch was composing poems about Gray's sickness, and wrote that his recent poems should collectively be called *"Cries of Our Occasions."* When Ray Gray died, on March 22, Lynch excused himself from his teaching obligations in Toronto to stay on in New York and attend at the funeral home. After the funeral service was over a group of them walked across town, with Spiers in his black funeral wear, carrying the casket spray, which included Dovima's hat and veil (Dovima was Gray's drag name). David Cohen, *"all multicoloured scarves,"* was holding Herb's arm. Etchy, an old friend of Ray's from Los Angeles who came to New York for the funeral, was trying her best to restrain Ray's two dogs on leashes. Lynch, *"sombre and overcoated,"* was two steps behind. *"A spectacle! It's over, it's beginning. I've cried and hugged for days."*

On the airplane back to Toronto, Lynch wrote another poem, "His Paintings," about Ray Gray. Robert Gildenhuys, whose Chicago friend had also recently died of AIDS, met him at the airport.

In San Francisco, debate over closing the city's gay bathhouses was heating up. Later, in fall 1984, authorities there would order fourteen bathhouses closed. Toronto's Public Health Department had already taken a quiet position against such a move, but ACT took pre-emptive action and prepared a press release opposing such a move in Toronto.[5] Public health officials, the press release noted, consider baths an important avenue of health education in the gay community. It quoted Fralick of the health department: "Gay baths are good for letting the gay community know what's going on with issues such as AIDS. Without them, we can't properly inform and educate gay men."

At the end of March Lynch travelled to Philadelphia for some academic meetings and managed to slip over to Camden to visit Walt Whitman's home—Lynch had his photo taken in Whitman's bed—and his nearby burial place. Poetry was flowing out of Lynch during this period—some of it recorded in draft form in his diaries. He taped into his diary a clipping from *The New York Times* about Léopold S. Senghor, poet and president of Senegal from 1960 until 1980. "It is difficult to imagine anyone more deserving of immortality than a man who has successfully blended poetry and politics," the article began. Making a comparison with himself, but recognizing his own vanity, Lynch made a notation: *"Ho! Ho! Ho!"*

In a March issue of *The Medical Post*, Health and Welfare Canada placed a four-page supplement on AIDS. It was a special edition of *Canada Diseases Weekly Report*, prepared by the National Advisory Council on AIDS. Aimed at health-care workers, the supplement noted that at the end of February Canada had seventy-five reported cases of AIDS, sixty-three of them in males. Of the total cases, twenty-two were in Ontario.

HIV had not yet been identified, and there was no test for exposure. The supplement advised doctors of a long list of "positive indicators" that a person might be at risk for having AIDS, including intravenous drug abuse, blood transfusions, the frequency of homosexual relationships, and the patient's status in these relationships (active; passive-receptive). The Council recommended a physical examination for lymphadenopathy, a visual examination of oral and rectal mucous membrane for lesions of Kaposi's sarcoma, thrush, and herpes, a neurological exam for possible cryptococcosis/toxoplasmosis infections, and several laboratory exams. When patients arrived in their offices showing "non-specific symptomatology" (fever, night sweats, weight loss, fatigue, and lymphadenopathy), doctors were advised to first rule out other possible causes such as tuberculosis, syphilis, and mononucleosis.

One night in mid-April, Lynch fell asleep reading in bed. When his new lover Stephen came in about three in the morning, he found Lynch in a night sweat, one of the warning signs of AIDS. Stephen stuck with him, though, and Lynch *"was happy to cuddle next to him all the rest of the night, and work nearby him as he slept in the morning."* The evening before Lynch had talked with Spiers, who was finding *"waves of The Death is Real, or He Isn't Coming Back,"* coming over him. A mutual friend from Fire Island, Vito Galiotto, had hanged himself after finding out he had Kaposis. Everyone in the community was fond of Galiotto. According to Spiers, they were all shocked by his death, but not particularly surprised because he was known for being both meticulous and fastidious.

AIDS Awareness Week, 1984

With its staff issues behind it, ACT began planning for a first-ever AIDS Awareness Week for Toronto, to be held in June. The inspiration was, in part, an "Aid AIDS week" held in New York City in 1983. Doug Bonnell in the health minister's office initiated a search for funding. Bert Hansen suggested that the week include a panel on women and AIDS and another one on "hemophilia and AIDS, why it concerns us all," which would include Bill Mindell. ("This was the golden age of co-operation," Mindell recalled.) Lynch had given Mindell the floor, at a January 5 ACT meeting with Norton, to make the case with the minister of health for comprehensive care clinics for Ontario hemophiliacs.[6] Mindell was representing the Ontario Hemophilia Society. Until that meeting, government bureaucrats had rejected the proposal, but Norton and Bonnell made sure it was approved. By then they knew that hemophiliacs would be hit by AIDS and would need to have adequate, knowledgeable care, Mindell said. "It was the only risk group where the only advice was to continue doing what you were doing."

As part of AIDS Awareness Week, U.S. journalist Nathan Fain, who had been reporting on the epidemic for the *New York Native* and *The Advocate*, was invited to come and speak about the recent French and U.S. announcements about, respectively, the lymphadenopathy-associated virus (LAV) and the HTLV-III retrovirus. In late April Dr. Robert Gallo had told a news conference in Washington that he had identified the virus that caused AIDS. At the time several scientists charged that he was stealing the spotlight from French researchers, whose LAV might prove to be the same as HTLV-III.[7] Indeed, investigators later determined that "Gallo's HTLV-III samples had a 99 per cent genetic similarity" to the virus that had been earlier identified by Dr. Luc Montagnier. It would appear that "Gallo had in fact 'discovered' Montagnier's virus."[8]

Also to be screened at AIDS Awareness week was *AIDS: After the Fear*, the second of two videos made by filmmaker and writer Michael Riordon for the University of Toronto's Instructional Media Services. The first video, *AIDS: A Challenge to Professionals*, available at the end of 1983, had featured several health-care professionals (including Bill Mindell and doctors Stan Read, Hillar Velland, and Randy Coates) speaking about AIDS, as well as Lynch talking about the social context of AIDS and the purposes of ACT. Near its end the video featured an interview with Peter Evans, who told the camera that his goal was to "go back to some normality" and resume his career.

After the Fear focused on the social context of AIDS. In it Hansen compared AIDS to cholera, noting that both epidemics aroused panic and hysteria, and primarily affected disadvantaged people. Cholera, he noted, diminished and disappeared before effective treatment was available. Jim Tennyson of ACT recounted how the organization was receiving telephone inquiries from fearful people asking if they should dismiss their Haitian housekeepers and babysitters.

For their part, Haitians were vigorously protesting the racism inherent in labelling their community a high-risk group, and had charged the city's Public Health Department with racism. The Mayor's Committee on Race Relations addressed the issue on May 15, with Lynch among the speakers. *"My hidden agenda, since that morass was inevitable quicksand, was to stay friends w/the Health dept, to try to show yet again that we're 'with' the Haitians, & to prompt the mayor to designate AIDS Awareness Week."* He had trouble judging the impact of his talk, he said. The last time he had spoken to a City Hall committee was eleven years earlier, and he enjoyed doing a little speech now. Although he had confronted the department, he and Mindell left the meeting together and had a friendly chat as they walked up University Avenue on *"a not-so-cool night, clear, full mooned."*

Lynch kept up a hectic pace of work and play during these months. On Monday, May 21, he told his diary that he "lurched home" at 4:30 a.m. after spending three hours "acid-wired" at the disco Stages. Two days later he spent the day at Erindale College catching up on correspondence for the *Gay Studies Newsletter*, a publication of the Lesbian and Gay caucus of the Modern Language Association and edited by Lynch from 1981 to 1990 (it was later known as the *Lesbian and Gay*

Studies newsletter). Lynch was feeling a flu coming on and he bowed out of an ACT meeting that evening. He took to his bed, and Stefan made him chicken soup for dinner. *"Perhaps I'm a superman, a real power to contend with, an intransigent force, in only one area: Stefan's inner future. That is a terrifying thought."* He also worried that Stefan would have his father to grapple with all through his life. *"He is now so warmly attached to me. So close."*

The next day Lynch headed to New York City with Stefan and Cam Lawford, a friend of Stefan's, in tow. Stefan, who'd been to New York before, was "proudly urbane" and his friend talkative and wide-eyed as they visited the Empire State Building and the World Trade Center, and then took the Circle Line Tour around Manhattan. They stayed for the weekend with Spiers, who, according to Lynch, was enduring his "pained grief" and glimpsing "the possibilities of sui-cide." On Monday Lynch took the boys to the Brooklyn Bridge. He must have told Stefan, who was twelve years old, that he wanted his ashes scattered on the East River near the bridge, because his diary recorded that Stefan said, *"I don't know how I'll get your ashes from here to the water. Perhaps a motorcycle along the roadbed below and a short stop . . ."*[9]

Toronto Mayor Art Eggleton had been slow to officially sanction AIDS Awareness Week, and ACT only received official notice of his endorsement on the Friday before the week was to begin, too late to use in the publicity. At ACT's June 4th press conference to announce the week, Lynch castigated the mayor for his "evasion of leadership" and "callous insensitivity." (He later wrote in his diary that he was "invigorated" by the attack, but allowed that it might have been an oversight that he didn't warn other board members of his plans.) The press conference featured an empty chair for the late Peter Evans—in part to honour him, in part because no other person with AIDS could be found to go public with the illness.

"AIDS Awareness week marks a transition in the public response to AIDS in Canada," Lynch told the press conference. "A year ago, we saw irrational fear and panic. Those responses have largely given way to a growing awareness of AIDS." The week's activities included four forums, eighteen speakers, and screenings of two videotapes—"the most comprehensive such effort to date in Canada," he said.

Lynch also praised the Toronto Department of Health and the Ontario Ministry of Health, which he said had set examples of enlightened public health leadership. He noted, though, that ACT had not yet received funding from any public health budget, and its applications for core funding from the province and the federal government had been rejected.[10]

The panel "Women Talking about AIDS" featured women's health activist Anne Rochon Ford, who spoke about the similarities between AIDS organizing and organizing around issues of women's health, with particular reference to DES (diethylstilbesterol), a synthetic estrogen that was given to women for over twenty years to prevent miscarriage—even though it was proven to be ineffective for that purpose. DES caused reproductive difficulties and in rare cases cancer. Rochon-Ford outlined a dilemma that would much later—about four years later—come into clearer focus for AIDS activists. With both AIDS and DES, she noted, money was desperately needed for research and education—and the source for the money was the government. An article outlining her talk stated:

> Thus it is hard for activists to make public statements against government agencies, even though they may have been partly responsible for exacerbating or prolonging those health problems. Along the same vein (don't bite the hand that feeds you), it is risky for both DES and AIDS activists to criticize the medical profession. For years, health activists have been questioning medical authority, have been fighting homophobia and sexism in the profession and have been encouraging us to lessen our dependence on doctors. However, the treatment of such serious health problems as AIDS, cancer and reproductive abnormalities requires expensive and sophisticated equipment. And in order to cure these ailments we need solid medical research. In short, we need doctors. Rochon Ford stressed that the healthy have privileges which they can address by fighting for better medical education and for the eradication of sexism and homophobia in the health care professions. She also encouraged gay men to learn from the work of the women's health movement to address their own needs.[11]

For its first eleven months, ACT had survived on private fundraising and the $62,415 federal job-creation grant that had come through in

June 1983. With that grant due to run out on June 30, the organization was facing a major financial crisis. At the eleventh hour, on June 27, board members were told that the province had come through with $30,000. MPP Susan Fish, who was instrumental in obtaining the money, asked that the contributing ministries (health and citizenship and culture) not be credited by name; and a July 3, 1984, ACT press release announced the grant as being only "from the government of Ontario."

Lynch stepped down from ACT at the end of June, to be replaced as chair by Tom Alloway, another University of Toronto professor. Lynch, who had been instrumental in establishing other community-based organizations, such as Gay Fathers, had performed true to style. He had helped to identify a community need, written about the problem in the gay media, been in on ground floor of establishing a new organization, and then, when the venture was fully launched, withdrew and left it to others to run.

He had steered ACT through early, and perilous, times. "We were headed for destruction," recalled Kossmann of those first six months of 1984. "As board chair, Lynch did a wonderful job, largely because of his diplomatic skills. He made everyone feel important, he made you feel like you were the only one in the room . . . and he was a real heavy lifter. He did so many practical things, like making deals with provincial ministers."

The day after the June 27 board meeting, Lynch came home to hear from Lewis that his white blood cell (T-cell) count was very low for the third consecutive month. Concerned about his health, Lewis had convinced his doctor to put him through regular blood tests.

Safe sex and lover juggling

That summer Lynch taught a university course, took care of Stefan (who stayed through the summer, and would live with his mother during the upcoming school year), and prepared for his coming sabbatical in New York City. He also wrote poems and sent them out to journals and publishers—fifty-one poems in all, sent to eight or nine journals. All of the poems were rejected, he reported to a friend. He also sent two collections of poems (provisionally titled "Nipples" and "Cries of Our Occasions") to two different publishers.

At Gerald Hannon's fortieth birthday on July 7, Lynch and Spiers performed a drag act and recited written-for-the-occasion verse at midnight. Stefan got drunk, and Hannon made a speech saying he "was grateful for such wonderful friends during his first 40, and hoped they'd be with him through his second."

A week later, Lynch went to a funeral for what he dubbed Toronto's first "ghetto-familiar" AIDS death. Mike O'Neill's funeral was *"the first AIDS rites for us here"*—meaning the downtown gay circle. *"It's the social event of the season,"* Lynch told Lewis. *"There're gonna be so many of these—everyone will be doing it—and this is the very first. I'm sure anybody who's anybody will be there."* Lynch also flew to Chicago for the July 20th funeral, in the suburb of Kenilworth, of his former father-in-law, Gail's father Hayden Jones.

Pride Day 1984—Sunday July 1—marked another notable change. ACT distributed free condoms. The city's Public Health Department, happy to further the cause, donated five hundred condoms, although ACT chose to tell takers that the condoms were from an anonymous donor. Lynch, and other leaders of ACT, had significantly changed their thinking since Pride Day 1983, when Harvey Hamburg was criticized for promoting condom use. But the shift towards condom use was happening, and now even a lover of Lynch's was insisting on them. *"He doesn't want to be fucked, and I am quite glad to be fucked, even with a condom!"* Still, the organization warned that condoms were not a guaranteed way to prevent transmission of the AIDS virus.

The gay community's acceptance of condom use came quite quickly, given that in general people find it notoriously difficult to change sexual practices. In article written six years later, Simon Watney observed that gay men *invented* safer sex "long before the identification of HIV or the widespread availability of HIV antibody testing in the west."[12] He noted that Michael Callen's 1983 primer, *How to Have Sex in an Epidemic*, had stood the test of time remarkably well and represented an approach to safe-sex education strongly in contrast with most government-funded initiatives, which might collectively be regarded under the heading "how to give up sex in an epidemic."

At a lunch date in early August with Bonnell, the health minister's executive assistant, Lynch and his co-conspirator "talked, delicately," about gays among Ontario's ruling Progressive Conservatives. Lynch came home to a telephone call from Lewis, who was off visiting friends in Burnaby, B.C. Lewis was experiencing "another Kaposi's panic," and seeking reassurance. Shortly after Lynch hung up the phone, Stefan returned from the YMCA. *"He lies beside me, holds my hand for a while, wishes I'd play volleyball with him sometime. My first, albeit silent reaction, No. My second, YES, THERE ISN'T MUCH MORE TIME. It occurs to me that my state may be Hep B-related . . . Still, in a moment this is my deathbed and I am looking long and unwaveringly in his eyes. As Mama did ours."*

Stefan began to fret about leaving Toronto, where he had spent most of his life and all of his school days. Lynch, meanwhile, had his upcoming year put in perspective by his friend Ed Jackson, who pointed out: *"You have before you a year in NYC, no responsibilities, a salary, no **demands** except your muse"*—to which Lynch replied, *"She's a tough one."*

On Stefan's last evening in Toronto, Lynch threw an early evening champagne party, inviting a few of his friends (Hannon, Jackson, Lewis) as well as Stefan's friend Jonathan Leonard and Barbara Klunder, the mother of another of Stefan's friends. Lynch and Lewis later took the two boys to the rotating restaurant at the top of the CN Tower *"for 2 and a half hours of tolerable food, a stupendous electrical storm, much talk."*

On the verge of leaving Toronto himself, Lynch was busy juggling two lovers and engaging in escapades such as meeting one (Barry) on the fire escape at a dance club where the other (Stephen) worked. *"For a heterosexual, this would make me a prime cad. For a homo, it **may** do the same . . . I want to be w/Barry, but I don't want to exacerbate Stephen's pain."*

As the newer affair heated up, Lynch recognized an intensity that went hand in hand *"with the imminent separation"* that seemed an inevitable part of that kind of relationship for him. The affair brought a *"holiday-time sense of time: just a day out of life."* He was already growing "antsy" under the conditions of a full-time passion. *"It's wondrous, it's torrid, he's a soul-grappling fuck and pre- and post-fuck*

*companion, but to engage more of life (with its letdowns and boredoms
and needed privacies) would require a really different set of assumptions. . . .
I want to be a long-term friend—to me, that's love—but don't feel that
this passion is adequate to propel that."*

Lynch agonized over his lover/juggling act, then admonished himself. On August 20, he was turning forty, beginning a new personal decade. *"No, Michael, begin the decade more firmly, God knows if you'll live it out . . ."* On the eve of his fortieth birthday, he faced an ethical dilemma with his new lover: *"I wanted to fuck him, but not w/o condoms. He wanted my fuck, & said condoms didn't matter, he really wanted me to come inside him (frustrated by my inability to come, to yield up & whimper in abandon). So I fucked him, & faked orgasm. He was happy, thinking I'd come, & I was happy, knowing I hadn't. Is there any better image for the possible utility of lies?"*

The next day Lynch was chewing over *"the adopted child's birthday question, annual wonderment"*—is she still alive, does she think of me?

One of Lynch's last tasks before leaving for his sabbatical year—he'd rented out his apartment—was tiding up his books and papers. He had stacks of uncompleted manuscripts around the place—on Wallace Stevens, a draft novel ("The Very Man"), poetry, and other writing. The mess reminded him, he said, of his greatest fear. He desperately wanted to complete and be remembered for a book.

Instead of throwing a fortieth birthday party, Lynch's friends gave him a going-away party. In his diary, he listed all forty-two guests. Among them was his new acquaintance, Bonnell of the health minister's office. A week later, as he prepared to leave the city, a photographer from *Toronto Life* magazine arrived to take pictures of 8 Ross for a spread that would appear in the magazine the next spring.[13]

New York City, 43 West 19th Street

Lynch's friend Herb Spiers lived and worked in a 4,000-square-foot loft, with a fifteen-foot-high ceiling, in downtown Manhattan at 43 West 19th Street. Spiers and Bernd Metz, his business partner and co-owner of the loft, were at the time publishing graphic novels and had boxes and boxes of them. Lynch, who had arranged to spend his sabbatical year living in the loft, picked a spot overlooking the street and created a room for himself with walls made of boxed books. It was, according to Spiers, "the most clever bedroom. The walls were over 8 feet high, with a curved entrance, windows. Utterly fabulous, utterly Michael."

Once settled in the city, Lynch began work on the life of the "sodomites" (homosexuals/bisexuals) in New York City from the 1830s to the 1850s. For background he read Paul Zweig's new biography of Walt Whitman: he thought the book was bad on the gay stuff, but good *"on the subtle transformations of hack journalist to genuine poet."* The story was *"a wish-come-true"* for Lynch, *"perhaps for my journalist wishing to become a poet. WW, the ultimate self-made man, did it. He did it! Can I? Probably not."*

But Lynch was also awash in present-day concerns and gossip. Richard Howard, a prominent poet and translator, had translated a work on AIDS by Parisian Dr. Jacques Leibovitch, Michel Foucault's doctor. In a phone conversation Howard told Lynch that the theorist had died of AIDS. Author Edmund White confirmed this to Spiers, adding that Foucault didn't want the cause of death known because it would undercut his work. But, according to Lynch, Howard insisted that Foucault *"would never have wanted it concealed; it's left groups who still think that to have AIDS is a moral condition rather than a virus."*

Courtesy of his friend Michael Brennan, who gave him the keys to his house in The Pines, Lynch was able to spend some quiet time on Fire Island. In a reflective mood, he told his diary that he walked the boardwalks *"less ponderingly than in 1982, less timidly than in 1981. More self-confidently than either of those years, more me, more sad, more whole, more simply grateful, more secure, more aware of the brink of the end."*

Dancing was one of Lynch's great passions. "Once he got into dancing there was just no stopping him," Spiers said. But there was more going on than just dancing. In a poem scribbled in his diary in mid-September, Lynch wrote: *"I danced as I danced two years ago, alive with love. I danced with gabbing Larry, receding Ray, needlepoint Vince, armoured Michael, a dozen unnamed others whom the virus thinks it has taken from the floor."*

During the fall Lynch researched, attended New York theatre, opera, and concerts, and maintained a busy social life. But through it all he showed remarkable discipline. After a late night out doing drugs and dancing Lynch would catch a few hours' sleep, rise early with his coffee, and get to work. "I used to be so amazed," Spiers said. "I'd say, Michael, how can you *think*?"

Old flesh and bones, and the rise of toxoplasmosis

By October 1984 AIDS was still much more prevalent in the United States (where 6,182 cases had been reported), but it was gaining ground in Canada. The 147 adult cases of AIDS reported in Canada as of November again indicated that the epidemic, while growing, was still about two years behind its Southern neighbour.[14] Near the end of November, Lynch received a letter from a very upset Alan Miller, who had just learned that librarian James Fraser had advanced KS and there was nothing that could be done. *"I grieve,"* Lynch said, *"but on a back burner."* His main reaction to the news was to get to the library, get his work done. *"I understand those anecdotes of scholars or lab scientists who won't leave their carrels to attend a colleague's funeral; the man who said 'let the dead bury their own dead.'"*

By that time one friend after another was falling victim to AIDS. Bob Marshall, who was known as "Mayor of The Pines" and had a pool at his Fire Island house, got sick in October. By November Marshall was in hospital with toxoplasmosis, a brain infection that is one of the devastating opportunistic infections that defines the onset of AIDS. Lynch and Spiers went to visit Marshall at St. Luke's Hospital, where they found a disturbing mixture of hallucinations and violent, physical words and actions—and, at least for a few moments, gentle, clear, logical conversation. The violence came from the hallucinations, Marshall told them the second day they visited, and he was being labelled psychotic. "It's strange to lie here on my deathbed having good friends come to visit," he would tell them, and then, the next moment, he would confuse dates (day, date, even year), time sequences, where he'd been. A sense of paranoia would emerge ("They've got dead bodies in every room here, Herb, and they've got a plot on me too"), or fantasy ("I'm not afraid of dying because I have got three lives and I'm just moving from one to another").

For Lynch, the apparent lucidity at moments felt like real contact, but he found it disturbing that those moments had no more "reality"—in terms of consistency, or endurance—than the other times—*"when what we said intelligently to each other one moment would be, in the next moment, as if never said at all. It made me not want to say anything, or to say anything, because it didn't matter, or, a moment later, wouldn't."*

The trip by train to the hospital and back *"was slow and filthy"* and hard on Herb, who had been helping Bob over the past six months. *"Herb was much reminded of Ray's deathbed today,"* Lynch wrote. *"Bob even said, at one point after talking of dying, 'You've had a lot to go through this year Herb.' Herb answered, 'So've you.'"*

Lynch travelled to Dunn in early December to visit his younger brother Pat and was annoyed when he wasn't woken up on Sunday to go to church. He wanted to go to church and make witness to their mother's presence—*"to her death, in a tie-and-suited son who comes and sings and stands, but passes over the host and will not close his eyes for any prayers."* He didn't know why it mattered, but it did, and half the reason for the trip to Dunn, he said, was to go to church that morning. *"A few more years and all the Alices and Agnes and Elizas and Marys who knew her will be gone, but while they're here I want to say—I come, I sit and stand, I sing in her place in her absence. Dorothy Lynch lives, and lives in me."*

Before leaving town, Lynch dropped into a senior citizens home to visit Mary Pridgen, his high-school math teacher, who was dying of cancer. Years earlier, he had visited her to show off his toddler son. Lynch told his diary that he saw in her face, half paralyzed by a stroke, the Mary Pridgen of twenty-five years earlier in her classroom and of sixty years earlier in her high-school yearbook. Mary, frustrated by not being able to read, explained that she was not interested in chemotherapy. She had lived a good long life and had no complaints. "I'll always remember you, Mike," she said as he was leaving.

"I love old flesh and bone," he wrote later. *"She was so alive and vivid to me in her voice as if she were demonstrating quadratic equations."*

Back in New York, he worried about congestion that he had been suffering in his lungs, and what felt like the onset of another flu. *"Naturally, I think immune deficiency. And when & where & how I'd end my life. I would not move to self-termination until an AIDS diagnosis was **fully** confirmed, but would then move A.S.A.P. before I'm incapacitated and in the hands of a doctor Hippocrates who won't respect the right to die."* He considered the options of dying in a hotel room, and leaving a note for whoever found him—apologizing and asking them to call his lawyer, Harvey Hamburg. Only his housemate Lewis would know of his plans in advance, and Lewis and Hamburg would be instructed to call Stefan, Gail, (his brother) Pat, Herb and Bernd, and *"anyone else they felt was appropriate."* He would, he thought, leave a general letter for friends and family and a special letter for Stefan.

A visit to a doctor a few days later, followed up by some X-rays, found him free of pneumonia and suffering only from an influenza virus.

Lynch celebrated Christmas 1984 in New York with Stefan, who came all the way from California, and Lewis, who came from Toronto. Afterwards, the three of them headed off for a special trip to Washington, D.C. Lynch was struck by Stefan's about-to-be-adolescent self, by a sudden vision of his son's adult shape and self. Lewis, meanwhile, demonstrated an "unaccustomed sweetness." That both pleased Lynch, and scared him. *"Does something in him know it's one last time together as a trio?"* Despite the doctor's assurances—and the lung X-ray results—Lynch continued to worry about his cough and the possibility that he might have PCP. But when he returned to New York from Washington, further test results showed no sign of immune weakness.

Lynch and Lewis shared a bed on the last night of Lewis's visit to New York, but Lynch was so nervous about the setup that he came home late, gave them both sleeping pills, and waited until his took effect before getting into bed. He then contrived not to touch Lewis all night long. He noted his own coldness, his strange resistance, his fear, the massing of contradictions. *"Yes! I want to love, be loved, give, be close, break out of a box, write it all beautifully, father and lover fully, say; No! I don't want to depend, to be weak, to be **part**, to yield my higher isolation, to receive love, to be done for, to be trapped."*

five

THESE WAVES OF DYING FRIENDS

"Uncap the rads and fill the room with fear."
— Michael Lynch, "Conspirators"

For Michael Lynch, 1985 would usher in a steady stream of illnesses, deaths, and funerals—at first in New York and later in Toronto. It was a bleak period in the epidemic; there were as yet no proven treatments and a mounting number of deaths. It all began promptly with the January 3 funeral of Bob Marshall, an event that offended Lynch: *"Friends gathered for Bob's funeral & were ignored, the rabbi paying all attention instead to his sister, who had ignored him."* Lynch had little tolerance for funerals and memorials at which vital aspects of the life of the deceased, such as sexual orientation, partners, and friends, were studiously ignored

Less than two weeks later he heard that another one of his New York friends, Blair Swain, was ill. Swain worked for Citibank and, with his partner Ken Calendar, had been exceptionally attentive when Larry Okin was dying. By happenstance, the evening after Lynch heard, most of his New York circle of friends converged on the dance floor at the Saint. They didn't talk about Swain's illness, but they were all thinking of it. Finally, after hours of dancing, Bruce Schentes danced over to Lynch—*"hugged me, burst into tears holding me, or holding on to me, saying 'I'm so scared.'"*

After visiting Swain in the hospital, Lynch ruminated on his changing response to illness and death: *"Even sitting in the bed by Blair—bald, sallow, skin-lesioned, utterly drawn & strengthless—I don't seem to believe it; or perhaps after several it just doesn't matter so much any more."* He thought about his mother, and grandmother, and their responses to death—so stoic, without much brooding or mourning. He wondered whether experiencing "first deaths" for a child or young adult meant mourning for all the deaths that are yet to come—*"as one might pre-pay one's taxes or hotel bill and not have to worry further."*

> *My response to Larry Okin's had a lot of this firstness, since I was less close to him than say to Ray or even Blair. Many of the eulogistic pieces I see in the gay press—as mine for Larry—share a quality of firstness . . . ordinary people, ordinary deaths. Who might now die that would derange me? Only—I guess—Stefan, Gail, because I live through it with Stefan, who can't be spared her (or my) death someday. Bill's. Maybe Herb's.*

Lynch took Swain's parents to lunch on the last Monday in January. He thought they were good and decent people, Christians who had more love than judgement. They were calm. He thought Blair should have come out to them years earlier. For many men, like Swain, developing AIDS was the catalyst for telling their parents that they were gay. Some parents were left reeling from the double revelation, but supportive, while others reacted to the news by washing their hands of their own children.

When Lynch visited Swain the day after his lunch with the parents, the two men discussed the design of the oxygen canister to which the patient was now connected—"so early high tech," Swain observed. He died several hours later, surrounded by his parents and friends. *"Rest in peace, Blair,"* Lynch told his diary. *"Your death differs from the others in that it's you, but also in that we're so **accustomed** now."*

In California, thirteen-year-old Stefan was settling into his new school. He telephoned at the end of January with news of a stellar report card. It was his first encounter with being given grades, because in primary school in Toronto he had attended an alternative school that had a policy of not dispensing marks. Stefan received all A's, except for a B in physical education. "I'm proud of me & I hope you are!" the boy enthused. Lynch felt his own work, meanwhile, was not going all that well. He was researching and documenting, at archives and libraries, what was known about male-male relationships in New York City in the nineteenth century, and he was thinking about writing his own biography of Walt Whitman.

Deciding to escape winter for a bit, Lynch flew to California in February to visit Stefan and Gail, Pat Bond (now separated from Gail), and friends in San Francisco. He found Stefan expressing feelings more readily than ever before and wanting as much as possible to do everything with his mother and father and him together. Gail, Lynch thought, was still sexually attracted to him, which made him uneasy. But he recognized his uneasiness as being associated with a sensation—close to fear, perhaps—that he had sometimes felt in the company of his mother, when he sensed that she was sexually teasing him. Bond, the performance artist, was "wracked with crisis" over turning sixty and facing career, income, and housing insecurity: *"a quivering, frightened 60."* Lynch subsequently began sending Bond small sums of money on a monthly basis, enough to allow her the odd luxury. It was a kind gesture, typical of a man who was well aware of his privileged position as a tenured professor. In New York Lynch was hanging around with many men wealthier than himself, but at home in Toronto he was one of the most well-off and secure of his *Body Politic*, activist, and artist friends. Lynch's friends in San Francisco, meanwhile, were into s&m. Lynch loved *"being tied up and allowed to go into my own squirming and whimpering and submission."*

Back in New York, Lynch learned that Richard Umans, Michael Brennan's partner, had died. "Uncap the rads and fill the room with fear," began the poem, "Conspirators," that he wrote in his diary in response to this and the accumulating AIDS deaths. The final version of this poem would later become Lynch's most widely quoted elegy to the toll of the epidemic. Lynch had not seen Umans when he was ill, and now had to struggle to cope with his death:

> *I tried, but couldn't imagine his decline and dying in any way that convinced me: I can't even picture him "pale" (as my poem said he was in Sept.) much less enervated and drawn, yellow or green, gasping for a last few days of breath. I can't, it won't **work** that way. I see Larry blind and feeble, I see Ray paltry and tubed, I see Blair bald*

*and semi-comatose, I see Bob deranged: and these visions, without interfering with my visions of them well, persuade, **convince** me they were ill. But Richard?*

How to cope with the unending deaths? *"You get embarrassed when someone dies before you've even heard they're sick,"* Lynch later observed.

In the following year Lynch wrote in his diary about sticking gold stars—like the ones his piano teacher used to affix beside titles of pieces that he had mastered—next to names in his address book of friends who had died. The entries were often crowded with additional telephone numbers, scribbled in pencil, mostly of hospital rooms. Lynch also wrote about placing the stars, like halos, over the heads of friends pictured in group snapshots, and sticking them on the tabs of file folders containing correspondence from now-dead friends.[1] In a poem about this, Lynch concluded:

> *At first each star went on with a struggle, like*
> *real stars combusting. Then habit [denatured?]*
> *rage, and the tang in each lick was a question*
> *aren't there some things you should never get used to?*
> *Now, paper stars go on with the ease*
> *of a meteor burning out. They mean*
> *you can put these aside now*
> *not to practice anymore.*

In New York Lynch resumed therapy with Sage Walker, who was now also living there. Lynch had first started working with her in the late 1970s, for counselling with Gail, and continued to see her for individual therapy for several years after that. In this pursuit he was unusual among his political activist friends, although both Lewis and Spiers were also clients of Walker's for a time. Much of the work, like the dreams he frequently recorded in his diary, centred on his early family life in Dunn and the loss of his father—indeed, the loss, even, of his father's name around the house. Lynch's relationships with his lovers and friends often had elements of the paternal. He publicly chastised his friends Ed Jackson and Gerald Hannon after they appeared in a photo accompanying a *Toronto Life* article in

April 1979, because they allowed themselves "to be turned into cold, arrogant, superior kids by *Toronto Life* photographers."[2] One of his friends referred to Lynch as "Daddy of us all." But he also suffered a tremendous fear of abandonment and an insecurity about how worthy he was to be loved. *"How do I say, casually, oh everyone's dying . . . & I'm not lovable or loved,"* he asked his diary, when agonizing over an inattentive lover.

At the same time, Lynch frequently expressed a great fear of being taken over, of losing himself in another. *"I need: But I don't take in very much, just want to turn in, into myself. O.K., it was my way of preserving my integrity when around a mother who would not let me be me."*

At Walker's suggestion, just before he left New York, Lynch attended a late April bioenergetic workshop in a town about an hour from the city. His response was (typically) divided. He wanted both *"to run away, to get the next bus to NYC"* and *"to be touched, held, gathered in to these people I'm eager to run from."*

The very next day, though, he recorded two insights:

> *Today's lesson explains a lot of all these years w/Sage, & despite my many little battles today I have a sense that I'll take it home. In the jargon, it's this: own up to your lower self. In my words: the key initial act of transforming/changing/growing involves accepting as my own every negative, destructive, dead, numb painful feeling I have. Even **treasuring** it. I hurt, but hoorah, **this** hurt is **mine**! I freeze, but this deathliness is **me**. I stonewall, but this is **my** wall.*

In a closing ceremony, workshop participants planted seeds and Lynch realized: *"All the gardens since Iowa, and this is the 1st time the seed (an ugly little marigold spike) was the 1st time I planted myself, identifying that in myself that I wanted to grow. My tears welled up, as so often in the past in church or the present w/music, & I had to cry, and cried hard . . ."*

As a sort of last fling in New York, Lynch applied to pose for some gay soft-core pornography. *"He found my age showing in my ass & rear waist, but took Polaroids frontally & I'm to call today to see if they'll 'use' me. Be bold, be bold, but not too bold, says WW [Walt Whitman]. I hesitate a bit but it seemd & seems a venture I must make. I do tingle & feel silly-gleeful at finally doing it."* It was the same feeling, he said, that he had experienced on his first trip to "the JAX." The New York Jacks, a group that met at the Mineshaft on Tuesday nights, was the city's hottest jerk-off club. With the fear of AIDS, mutual masturbation clubs and parties had come into vogue.

Lynch was scheduled to return to teaching summer courses at Erindale in mid-May, and his last week or two in New York was a social whirl, with a farewell party thrown by Bruce Schentes and David Cohen, and a constant stream of coffee, lunch and dinner dates, and gift-giving. *"If I **can** leave New York, I can die, leave life,"* he wrote, melodramatically, in his diary. Lewis arrived to "provide overlap" and accompany Lynch home to Toronto, a city that he described, on his return in early May, as "bovine." At a coming-home dinner, his friend Robert Trow told him, "You don't have to pretend to be glad to be back. *We* don't like it here."[3]

But within a few days, Lynch had started teaching his university courses and observed that his *"NY lenses were off"*—he could see and enjoy Toronto's virtues.

Saying yes

During his nine months in New York, Lynch had experienced a steady stream of AIDS deaths. By the time he arrived back in Toronto, the epidemic locally—deemed now to be just a year and a half behind the United States—was gaining force. The number of deaths was mounting. But there was also love. At a party on Saturday night, May 18, Lynch met Sam Nirenberg, and they busily cruised each other. Nirenberg, twenty-eight, was still at Lynch's house the next morning when John Ward telephoned and announced that he wanted to die there. The request was a bit odd because Ward, a thirty-four-year-old medical doctor and research pathologist who had PCP, was more of an acquaintance than a friend. But Lynch did take him in at 8 Ross Street for a couple of weeks, although refusing a long-term arrangement. *"A haven I've offered, but a hospice, no. John's been eager to turn me into a full companion as well as a host. No."*

While he could say "no" to Ward, Lynch could think of no reason for resisting Nirenberg. By early June, when the younger man headed to Italy for a holiday, the two had declared themselves lovers. Perhaps it was the result of all the work he'd done in therapy in New York, perhaps he was ready, or perhaps this was the right person at the right time. Whatever it was, Lynch allowed himself to fall in love with Nirenberg, allowed Nirenberg to fall in love with him, and allowed himself to accept that love in an unprecedented way. Since his intense, three-year-plus relationship with Bill Lewis had ended, Lynch had gone through several relationships and many sexual liaisons. But this one was different. *"He is indeed your lightbulb, beaming and illuminating,"* Lynch wrote. *"Everyone around you likes him— Herb, Michael* [Jorgensen], *Bill, Gail."* Stefan was back in Toronto for the summer, and he too, Lynch noted, had fallen in love with Sam, and Sam with Stefan. *"Sex is wonderful & shows signs of self-renewal even this early on—you doubt some thing ('I only want to make you happy'—is this possible w/o self-loss?). But so much else pushes in like roots . . . Blow this one and you'll regret it for a long time."*

In early June Lynch was back in New York, presenting a paper to the Hofstra History Conference on the research done during his sabbatical. His was the best-attended session, and an editor at Syracuse University Press inquired if Lynch would be writing a book. Earlier, he had received an enthusiastic response from the University of Chicago Press to a book proposal based on his work on what he was calling the "Age of Adhesiveness." But he became less keen when Chicago offered no advance and no contract until the book was delivered. At the same time, thoughts of writing inspired worries about mortality: *"Every AIDS report—even of Rock Hudson!—strikes out all the clocks in the house and burns the calendars."*

On the domestic front, Lynch and Nirenberg became a team at taking care of funeral arrangements. When Larry Webb, the roommate of one of Nirenberg's best friends, died of AIDS in early August, the new couple took care of things. When they went to Mount Pleasant Cemetery to get a plot, they both wondered, "Why do we have to do all this?" Nirenberg said. "But Larry was estranged from his family. And we knew how to do it."

Just over a week later, Lynch recorded a dream:

I am watching a huge steam shovel dig out a deep hole in front of my house, part of the renovations. The thing suddenly slips and slides into a precarious position: momentarily it will crash into the excavation and crush the three people running it. As it hangs there, and we watching it grip our chests with fear, the 3 operators—one a woman—ease out of the cockpit. There is no way for them to escape; they will be crushed. All together, as if by long prearrangement, they look at us and leap to their deaths. We wonder at their heroism.

Stefan, now taller than his father, spent his summer practising tennis and taking lessons. From time to time, he told his father to smile. *"I don't smile much these days, am not unhappy but find myself looking at smilers and thinking, 'oh, people do.' All amusement seems, while inoffensive, deprioritized."* Lynch wrote that passage while on holiday with Stefan and Lewis in Quebec City. Lewis was ill and unsociable, and Lynch, feeling enormously fatigued, often met his son's enthusiasm with sourness. It was quite unlike the upbeat and companionable Washington trip that the three had shared the previous Christmas— the trip that Lynch feared would be their last together.

What did have priority for Lynch was his academic writing. He was hoping to make his mark with a book on his "Age of Adhesiveness," followed by the biography of Walt Whitman. In the fall he made a pilgrimage to visit Gary Wilson Allen, a Whitman biographer who had retired from teaching at New York University in the late 1960s. Allen, who lived with his wife Eve in Oradell, New Jersey, took Lynch to his attic study to talk. He told the younger man that in his work he had reached a point where he thought it safe to assume that whatever else he learned about Whitman's background would confirm what he already knew. That was when, he said, he began writing.[4] But teaching, relationships, and constant deaths interfered with Lynch's own writing plans.

Nirenberg moved into 8 Ross Street at the beginning of November, an event that for Lynch prompted memories of a much-loved aunt and uncle, Mary Helen and Mac:

This is a honeymoon. This is a form of happiness in the frame of "marriage." Possibly that is why M and MH come to mind, bubble up like a hot spring now. For of all the marriages I knew, growing up and longing for one as my source of happiness, their's alone seemed to have it. How I adored MH. Romantic, fussing over house and husband as a romantic lead should be (marriage seemed irrelevant, they were in love), a stager of intimate dinner a deux and of vacations a deux . . . I wrote her often as a kid. Third grade, I remember. She and Mac were ideal.

As he wrote that, Lynch realized how his idealization of that couple must have grated on his mother, struggling to raise two sons while her husband was in and out of alcohol treatment centres.

Near the end of November, John Ward asked Lynch and Eilert Frerichs, a United Church chaplain at the University of Toronto, to help him plan his funeral and memorial gathering. Lynch was gripped by Ward's "calm and even serenity." He talked to him about how he would want to be remembered. *"It is the second time on a Sunday night I've been pacified, centered by a quiet time with him."*

Bumfucking, swallowing cum, and organizing

The urban gay community was "battered, embattled, beleaguered, fearful, mourning, longing, and tired," Lynch wrote that fall. "We are hardly the first community to face suffering and death on a large scale. . . . But we are having to learn a lot about terminal illness, unspeakability and death awfully fast."[5]

It had been more than two years since Lynch had written any major articles for *The Body Politic,* but on Monday, November 24, he sat down and wrote ten pages on AIDS and obscenity while eating a dozen chocolate chip cookies. He liked the feeling of starting and finishing something, *"the neglected pleasure of journalism."* The article was published under the headline "Saying It: When we shy away from 'dirty' words, we lose the only language in which we can speak frankly of our sex and how to keep it safe. Michael Lynch on the need to reclaim our delicious obscenity."[6] In "Saying It" Lynch managed, as he had in his past journalism, to describe and assess a disturbing situation, and point to a way through the quagmire. He had decided that mourning had its phases, the last of which was action, and that unless mourning turned to action "its special blessing" would disappear. He told the readers: "Your experience may overlap with some parts of this, may be different. But we probably share a deep paralysis of fear and mourning." Authorities and the mass media, he said, were glossing over the truth about how AIDS was transmitted, were fuzzy about safe sex, and even censored explicit language. Canada Customs had censored safe-sex advice in an issue of *Blueboy*, a U.S. publication, prompting Lynch to observe that in Canada, "Dirty words are more dangerous than risky sex. Such puritanism has always been deadening; in this case it could turn out to be deadly as well."

Lynch argued that a recent Toronto documentary, *No Sad Songs* (by director Nick Sheehan), showed a community "badly in need of a vivifying current, a shock to action." It would be another two years before the Toronto gay community was driven to the kind of political action that Lynch envisioned.

With lives at stake every day, the prevailing lack of clarity and misinformation about transmission became deeply serious problems. "When I'm asked these days what are the chief modes of transmission of AIDS, I reply: every broadcast and newspaper article that is not offensively specific about swallowing cum when sucking dick or bumfucking without a condom." The gay community must insist on speaking for itself, using its own vocabulary:

> Our arousal will come in conjunction with our words. We will at times lay aside our fear and mourning and revivify our language. . . . When we come back to our obscenity . . . we will bring back to our culture a specificity, and thus a safety, that has been lost. If they take away our language, it is easier for them to take away our marginal bars and baths. If they take away those because someone says they're health hazards, we lose a particularly promising lab for developing a new safe sex culture.

The article was written a few months after a briefing note from Ontario Ministry of Health bureaucrats advised against funding the AIDS Committee of Toronto for a number of reasons, including the AIDS brochures that ACT was creating for the gay community. "We think it is inappropriate that such *propaganda* be printed with public money," the briefing note stated.[7] Included was a copy of the "parachute" brochure, produced by ACT in mid-1984. The brochure included specific safer sex advice, and used formal as well as colloquial language—for example, "Passive anal intercourse (getting fucked)." Perhaps the bureaucrats were offended by the language, perhaps they were put off by statements such as: "AIDS has been exploited by some people to resurrect old guilts about being gay. But the arrival of the AIDS agent in North America a few years ago was simply bad luck. Gay sex is a good and healthy thing, and AIDS does not prove that it isn't." Curiously, given the attitude towards the brochure, another reason cited for not funding ACT was that it was "*duplicating the work of the City of Toronto Health Unit and the Provincial Advisory Committee on* AIDS, *both of which are funded by the province, in providing educational material.*"[8] The bureaucrats, clearly, wanted to have it both ways—it's obscene; it's just duplicating other efforts.

In the years between 1984 and 1988—after the AIDS Committee of Toronto was created and before the activist group AIDS Action Now! emerged in the city—there was steady development across Canada of gay community and other service organizations to deal with the epidemic. AIDS Vancouver was born in the spring of 1983, after a group of gay men sponsored that city's first public forum on the illness. The Manitoba Gay Coalition began distributing pamphlets about AIDS and held an AIDS forum in August 1983. In January 1984, the Montreal AIDS Resource Committee, a division of Gay Montreal Association, was founded, and near the end of that year Halifax's gay community created a Gay Health Association to respond to AIDS. By 1985 the Gay Alliance Towards Equality in Edmonton had set up an AIDS Network in that city.[9] The year 1986 saw the formation of the Vancouver PWA Coalition and the Toronto PWA Foundation, as well as the Canadian AIDS Society (CAS), a government-funded organization established to represent AIDS service organizations in the country. CAS had been conceived at the May 1985 first national conference on AIDS ("All Together/Tous ensemble") held in Montreal, funded by Health Canada. In 1987 the federal government established a Federal Centre for AIDS. But with the noteworthy exception of the Vancouver PWA Coalition, there was still little overt political activism around AIDS.

The moment of death

With the 1985–86 holiday season approaching, Michael Lynch was sitting through part two of a Mendelssohn Choir performance of the "Christmas Oratorio" when he spotted a dark red spot on the back of his right thumb.

> *Noticed it earlier, but during Bach's meditations on death . . . I became convinced it was a KS lesion. I'm tight chested now over it, will watch for several days before checking with an MD . . . I think of finishing things up, of farewells, of secrecies, it is hard, just now, not to point out to Sam or Bill, but it is—appears—so real I won't.*

He endured two days of immobilizing worry and self-absorption. At a university seminar the next evening, he was *"almost taciturn, as a wounded future is."* Then he went to the doctor, who told him it was not a lesion. *"Now I come back into living awhile, but feel very tired."*

Six days later, on December 17 at 6:28 p.m., John Ward died, with Lynch at his side. It was the first time that Lynch had been present at the moment of death. He noted that he had missed his mother's death, his grandmother's, Ray Gray's (by a minute), Blair Swain's. He saw it as an important experience, a crucial experience. It reminded him of how, when he was in his late twenties, his mother, stepfather Charles Lee, and brother Pat had begun talking to him about money (the family's, their own), and he knew that he was at last an adult.

> *Something like that today; having seen John breathe the last breath, I'm more than familiar with the stranger. Gradually it sinks in: John isn't here. Gradually, a vacuum arises . . . The energy is dispersed, dispersing . . . His deep wide glaring mad eyes. The two big veins on his forehead, alone between skull & skin. Frenzied hands and kicking restless legs. Foaming mouth at the end. Congested throat, trying to speak like a drowning person . . . Body angled like The Man w/The Blue Guitar (what's Picasso's title!), on one side. Eyes dead before the last breath, yet refusing to close after it.*[10]

Lynch took a strong dislike to Ward's father, a prominent Toronto businessman, and once again railed at the hypocrisy of a formal funeral, at which the words gay and AIDS were not to be spoken.[11] He confronted the father on that omission, stayed away from the full service, and even refused the parental "smoothings-over" at the funeral home visitation. Lawrence Bennett, another friend of Ward's, was astounded at Lynch's insensitivity. "At the wake, the father was stricken and not a well man," Bennett remembered. Ward "admired his father and talked frankly to him about being gay," Bennett said, adding that Ward's parents and sister didn't hesitate to come to the gay community memorial that Ward himself had planned.

Lynch, increasingly concerned about his own health, noted in his diary that Stefan had declared that *his* fear about AIDS was lessened: "Since you've been with Sammy I don't worry."

Immediately after Christmas, Lynch flew to New York City to the American Historical Association meeting to deliver his paper "The Age of Adhesiveness: Male-Male Intimacy in New York City, 1830 to 1880."[12] The paper argues that the city had an extraordinary sexual freedom during that period, a freedom that ended when reformists, the press, and the medical profession, having tackled the evils of prostitution, turned their attention to sodomy and other acts. Lynch was nervous about delivering the paper, which was still in an unrevised state. It was the same anxiety that he felt before any new audience—like his first presentation, on Gerard Manley Hopkins, to the Gay Academic Union, his first Modern Language Association paper, or the history conference in Hofstra the previous summer. *"I think of everything I don't know and anticipate a direct question from the floor on it."*

AIDS and *The Body Politic*: A language for management

In January 1986, *Body Politic* collective member Rick Bébout wrote a five-page memo "to all those interested in *TBP/Xtra* and AIDS," critiquing AIDS coverage in the publications and trying to chart a "more coherent and conscious approach" for the coming year.[13] *The Body Politic's* "line" on AIDS, Bébout argued, was very different from the approach taken in the U.S. gay media. In particular, the Canadian newsmagazine had been consistently sceptical of scientific and media authority and had emphasized the need to resist panic and hysteria both within and beyond the gay community. It had asserted the need to seek information on which the gay community could make informed judgements about sexual practices. Most recently (perhaps with a tip to Lynch's article "Saying It" in that very same issue), the paper had argued for "the need to preserve what is best and most distinctive about gay erotic culture in the face of a disease which apparently threatens its very roots." Speaking for the collective, Bébout stated, "We have in fact been following some of the most basic tenets of gay liberation as we understand it (or at least as I understand it): that we must take the power to *define* ourselves, *organize* ourselves, and *create* for ourselves a space in which our distinctiveness can flourish."

But Bébout also elaborated what he saw as the shortcomings of the newsmagazine's approach: that it had been short on both the kind of practical information that people needed to make "calm informed" decisions and on "any solid understanding of how people respond to this information when it appears, and why." He continued:

> This is a failing I believe we share with almost everyone involved in AIDS work, and which I suspect is the legacy of a gay movement always more comfortable defending the right to sexuality than in coming to grips with the practice of sexuality. . . what people actually *do* and what it *means* to them.

Ironically, he said, the gay liberation movement had not taken "our own sexuality and the erotic culture we've built around it seriously enough . . . nor has the politics and theory (as opposed to the social service aspect) of the movement taken seriously enough how ambiguous and painful that sexuality and that culture can be for many people involved in it."

In the following months *The Body Politic* tackled some of the issues Bébout raised. For example, Bébout himself wrote "The Quandary of Advice," published in the May 1986 issue. The article explored the evolution of advice about preventing AIDS and offered that the "single, simplest, and I hope most effective safe sex advice is 'If you fuck, use a rubber.'"

In the new year, in February 1986, Lynch and Nirenberg went to San Francisco and Los Angeles for a holiday. Lynch was happy, but puzzled: *"I love him, but I'm so unused (old theme) to loving **when I am also loved** that I've no skill at it. Absence, even of a night, clarifies this. We fit together in so many ways, so well, that I'm puzzled by the lack of puzzlement. Loss has been my métier, in solitude, & now I need no fear/welcome it: he's here for a long stay."*

Alan Miller's partner Graham (Gram) Campbell was diagnosed with PCP in March, and by the beginning of April his illness was moving quickly. *"But we hope it will not succeed yet,"* Lynch wrote. AIDS was continuing to strike at close range. Don Briggs, a doctor who had been active in Gays in Health Care in Toronto, was diagnosed with AIDS. Late in March Lynch had visited a New York hospital to see Robert Meadows, an actor friend of Ken Calendar's. On April 2 Gail delivered news that a friend of hers and Pat's had the disease. Bill Lewis, meanwhile, was sure he had ARC (AIDS-related complex) because he was having a recurrence of herpes every few days instead of once a month. *"All his paranoias and hypochondrias converge like Spanish grandmothers at mass. Whatever the basis for his fears. . . the possibility of WHL [Lewis] with AIDS struck me for the 1st time and darkened. Four cases of people I know have come to light in the last **week**, so a period of apprehension is timely."*

In mid-May Spiers telephoned from New York to say that Steve Goodman was in hospital with AIDS. Goodman, who liked to be known as "Go go del Rio Goodman," was a Fire Island friend, an airline steward, and aspiring writer. *"I'm not strong, & have moments of fear, resignation,"* Lynch wrote later that day. One such moment had come a couple of nights earlier, when he found himself reading Whitman's "When Lilacs Last in the Dooryard Bloom'd," a poem he hadn't looked at in years. The poem had been written as an elegy for President Abraham Lincoln, but Lynch was struck by the sense that it could serve as a common elegy for so many people who had died—and he *"wondered about the elegy for all of us I'd like to write some day."*

Lynch and Nirenberg decided to head out that weekend for New York and Fire Island. The morning after they arrived, Lynch and Spiers went to visit Goodman at the New York University Hospital Co-ops. Then they crossed the drive to visit Bob Meadows.

> We held his hand and both of us (men of experience now in these matters, you understand) wondered if each irregular rattling breath was his last. A chest-thumper therapist asked us—and his brother and mother—to step outside, & in 3 or 4 minutes her ministrations roused him, then killed him. He was green, graygreen, and stringy-haired, & we held his hand again as it began to cool.

Meadows's mother, who had been chased from his side as he died, was "heartbroken and livid," Spiers recalled. Lynch and Spiers took a cab to collect Ken Calendar and bring him to the hospital.

"No diminishing, no denying, no diversion," Lynch wrote. "It's a network of disfigured memories, of dying, of suffering unto death, of fear of dying. (This little congestion in my lungs, is it PCP or TB? These mild but recurrent night sweats of late, this long fatigue, are they symptoms too like Steve's to lead to another diagnosis?) I have a sense that I'll get AIDS but that I'll be one of the first for whom medical discovery comes in time, to be saved, restored, to be a survivor . . . "

After the funeral for Meadows, Lynch wrote:

> We gathered together around the round oak table
> at Bruce and David's. We had gathered
> like this before. But did you notice?
> Michael said later. This time we didn't need
> the leaf?

Nirenberg spent the May weekend on Fire Island. He was having increasing difficulty with AIDS, with being so constantly reminded of its toll. Lynch had been suffering from night sweats for two years. On May 21 he told himself that it could be related to hepatitis B, to subclinical HIV.[14] "It need not be a sign of AIDS. Yet I wake to wet sheets and start plans to die."

Fear of AIDS and the deaths of the past years began to take their toll, leaving Lynch exhausted and depressed. For years Lynch had relied on Dalmane (a benzodiazepine prescribed to quiet anxiety) to combat insomnia. In early June, a doctor started him on Sinequan, a major antidepressant. That May weekend, Sam and his friend Jack went "out touring" and Lynch remained behind:

> *exhausted, bleary-eyed, thinking of death: of Bob turning green with his long thin stringy hair, of Blair suppurating, of Larry blind and skeletal of . . . Of me, exhausted and bleary-eyed. Should we not complain, self-pity, wish for death? Everyone dies, or many have died young. Who am I to wish for better? What entitles **me** to friends who grow old, and die, or die young in accidents rather than over 2 years? Richard Umans sits there on the other sofa, but I do not make out what he is telling me. No secrets beyond the grave. I could curl up now and shut out the world & shrivel away, and when Sam & Jack returned there'd be only a leaf and a memory. How many of those who've come to my parties would come to my funeral, and would it matter, what would it matter?*

While he was on his sabbatical in New York, Lynch had met with Australian writer Dennis Altman to talk about the experience of AIDS in Canada. Lynch's review of Altman's landmark 1986 book *AIDS in the Mind of America* was in the June issue of *The Body Politic*.[15] He dubbed it the "best book to date" in tackling organizational responses to the epidemic and debates over issues such as research funding, bathhouse closing, blood testing, and the role of gays in policy formation. Indeed, he credited Altman with creating "a new 'subject' which future writers will be unable to ignore: the social construction of the epidemic." But Lynch found fault with Altman's academic distance from his subject. He believed strongly that writers should not approach cultural history by means of "mollification and self-distancing," that writers should not take up a stance of intellectual detachment as the only alternative to "fear and hatred." "I don't think that gay life in the United States today, embroiled as it is in all sorts of full-blooded vibrancies, can be understood through a bloodless prose."

In a personal letter of reply to the review, Altman agreed that the book had a certain coldness. "It was both an intellectual and an emotional decision to be analytic rather than emotional. I think I was almost too successful," he wrote. Altman patiently explained that he faced the problem of "how to express the awfulness of what is going on without falling into the trap of seeming to be just another hysterical panic-monger." What Lynch referred to as "a cold mask of rationality" was "in part a strategy to demand attention from those looking for excuses to discount what we have to say. But only in part, for I would be dishonest if I denied that the 'coldness' of the book is also in part my own strategy for surviving these times."[16]

Stefan graduated from junior high in San Rafael on June 12. That was also the date for Toronto's AIDS vigil, and in preparation Lynch jotted down the names of the fourteen men he knew who had died of AIDS: Richard Umans, Ray Gray, Blair Swain, Bob Meadows, John Ward, Michael O'Neill, Vito [Galiotto], Bob Marshall, Joey Giusti, Larry Okin, Dale Olson, Peter Evans, Larry Webb, Don Bell. *"Others? They don't come to mind just now. But I'll leave room."* Lynch did not think much of the vigil. *"The speakers spoke of loss and things like: holy places, First Corinthians, faith (in doctors and technicians!), community, support, thanks, and remembrance. All hollow words, to me, but the last."* One speaker apparently said that he couldn't say what was in his heart. Another speaker, *"as correct and easy, spoke of the 'fellas' who had died, and also the 'women,' the fellas and the women."* What was particularly bad, Lynch thought, was the "social workereze" that provided *"a language for management: grief work, caring, sharing."* The speakers *"calmed deadened the gathered crowd with words like blankets: soft, restrictive."*

> *Manage your fear and grief, they said, fit it into these forms, let it Build Community. But words like that—I use them too—will never build community like the one* [an obscenity] *that a passerby shouted. It galvanized us all. . . . Did you see queers behind the microphone? Or hear words that wake the blood . . . Did you hear anything but condom language—verbal "safes" to halt the spread of dangerous thought?*

Lynch then took himself to task for retreating from activism, for quitting rather than fighting. But a week later he wrote his signature poem, "Cry"—which, he said, *"came out of the despair and chaos of the last few years & weeks, & brought me with it."*[17] It concluded with the line "we . . . will not endure these waves of dying friends, without a cry." The act of writing it was transformative: *"My world is an enchanted one: I am still under the spell of 'Cry.' I don't feel that I made*

it, but that it made me. It made me a poet, or, rather, a poem. It is the
maker, I am the poem, the thing made." He said that for the first time
he had no self-doubt in giving a poetry reading at the next Modern
Language Association meeting, or at sending a poem off to poet
Richard Howard. Stefan's arrival back in Toronto for the summer
also lifted Lynch's spirits, but he felt his relationship with Nirenberg
was beginning to crumble.

Bill Lewis attended the Second Annual International AIDS Conference in Paris at the end of June 1986. The conference revealed the
scope of the emerging AIDS tragedy in Africa, without announcing
any breakthroughs in general. By the end of the week, Lewis was
writing in his diary, "My nodes ache as they have increasingly with
every presentation of the conference, every presentation of biological
and epidemiological gloom." He heard that 30 per cent of antibody-
positive gay men were dead within six years of the initial exposure;
that 30 to 60 per cent of gay men with lymphadenopathy were dead
within five years of the onset of the illness; and that there was "every
indication that it's a continuing irreversible phenomenon for all
infected."

One day, Lewis wrote, just after the session where he had first
heard the lymphadenopathy figures, he was trying hard to keep from
sobbing as he thought about himself and his friends and their possible deaths. A sexy, "close-cropped" man in his late twenties smiled
and approached him and started a conversation.

> As this man chatted me up, I brightened and could feel myself
> once again engage with the here and now. He was an American,
> now in Germany, he said. I asked if he were a post-doc—he looked
> somewhat confused and answered that he was with the US Army
> and was sent to the conference to help with the coordination of
> screening of records and personnel for HIV exposure. I asked how
> he felt about that (TAG[18] would be proud of me)—he answered that
> he loved Paris and didn't mind at all having to attend the confer-
> ence. Angry, finally I restated my question—"no, how can you jus-
> tify carrying out a screening program to victimize gay men?" He
> proceeded to give me the reasons, so confident, so American—I
> remember beginning to tremble inside. He reminded me that
> there were lots of gay men in the military, just that they were offi-
> cially not practising sexually—his eyes twinkled ever so subtly. I
> felt rage then, but impotent and bottled, and I turned and walked

away heaving. Tonight I joined Randy [Coates] and Mary [Dr. Mary Fanning] at a table with a man and a woman. Introductions, she says I'm Dr. _____ from the Public Health Service. Randy quipped, the *US* Public Health Service?[19]

On August 4, Steve Goodman died in New York. He was thirty-seven years old. Just before his death he asked for a beer and got it. When a nurse offered him a sedative, a chance to sleep, he asked, "Now what y'all got?" It hadn't been that long since Blair Swain had died, in Steve's arms. Lynch remembered Steve telling Blair's parents, "You've gained a dozen sons,"at Blair's funeral. Steve's words were *"so accepting & profound & unpretentious,"* Lynch said. *"How impossible, that Ray & Larry & Steve & Blair are all gone! And how impossible, that we go along with these deaths. For what else is there to do?"*

Immersed as he had been with dying and death among his gay friends, Lynch found the heterosexual world to be an alien place. At a straight party in downtown Toronto, he chatted with several women, and on his way home he started to think about the size of the impasse. *"They all still expect, assume, rely on themselves and their friends, with the odd exception, living a long time . . . I really don't **expect** more than a few more years, I realized on the way home."* As he was about to go to sleep that night, Lynch was afraid of another night—it would be the third in a row—of heavy sweats, of "clammy sheets" and frequent bedding changes.

In mid-September 1986 Lewis accepted a tenure-track job at the University of Toronto. *"Think of the security that offers!"* Lynch enthused. Meanwhile Lynch, the already tenured professor, was featured in a New York-based porno magazine when the photos that had been taken during his stay in that city were published.[20] (It was his first, but not his last, foray into becoming a porn star. There was also a spread of nude photos of him in the June 1988 issue of *Mandate*.)

Testing positive

The test for HIV had become available in Canada in the fall of 1985, but many in the gay community, and some AIDS doctors, advised against testing for several reasons. There was no treatment available for those who did test positive and, since it was recommended that all gay men practise safer sex anyway, tests results would not in themselves be altering behaviour. As well, there was the possibility that a positive test result in a person's medical records would jeopardize an application for life insurance, or an immigration procedure, not to mention employment, accommodation, and even friendships. Dr. Philip Berger told *The Body Politic* that he was completely opposed to the test. "It has zero public health benefit. The civil rights of patients have to be the paramount factor."[21]

In any case Nirenberg decided to take the test, although he backed into it by telling his doctor that he would like to know the results but would go crazy waiting for them. His doctor, according to Lynch, took that statement as a request for him to do the test surreptitiously, which he did. The test turned out to be negative.

Lynch, meanwhile, continued to think about his "Adhesiveness" book, hoping for the time to work on it: "*. . . would like to live into my seventies in good health & get some things done, NOT NOT NOT NOT die earlier than that (I'm too old, someone said, to die young)."* He didn't tell Nirenberg, but just over a month after the younger man's test results came in, Lynch decided to take the test.

In early November he wrote to Gail to tell her he was "out of AIDS politics." There was a national conference coming up in Toronto the following week—"Action/Direction," the Second Annual AIDS Conference (the first, "All Together/Tous ensemble" was held in Montreal in May 1985)—and he refused an invitation to make a "rabble-rousing address" to it. Featuring Harvard medical historian Allan Brandt as a keynote speaker, the event would be the founding conference for the Canadian AIDS Society, with the first board of directors being elected. But Lynch told Gail that after five years of "constant fret," he was glad to be out of the worry of AIDS politics, even though "we have one acquaintance hanging on at TGH [Toronto General Hospital]." He was delighted to have the politics out of his mind, "however much that is an evasion—it is a welcome and healthy and productive evasion from the depression I've lived through. Still no report on my HIV test, I'll let you know when I get it."[22]

On Remembrance Day Lynch recorded in his diary that his relationship was over. Nirenberg had received a job offer in Vancouver, at a considerable increase in salary, and had decided to take it. *"What has he given me? Energy & light, first, just sheer amused delight, and— second—a sense that I **can** be loved. The most magical memory is of his holding on to me at night & saying, 'Michael, I love you.' Perhaps next time I can say that in return more readily."*

Nirenberg, many years later, recalled that part of the appeal of the job in Vancouver was the opportunity it provided to escape from the devastation of AIDS. "When I think of my time with Michael, so much of it was spent going to hospitals and funerals," he said. Both of them were caregivers, good at visiting people and helping out. Nirenberg was twenty-nine years old when he headed west, but he had already lost more than a dozen friends to the epidemic. Of course, people were also dying of AIDS in Vancouver, but not people he knew, not his old friends.

Lynch received the results of his HIV test on November 14. He had tested HIV-positive. The result came as no surprise, as he admitted, because he had already been thinking about the possibility of himself as an infected person for some time, though he had been hoping otherwise. But now his mind began to focus in a different direction. The new knowledge made a difference: *"intensifying the sense of transience, of tomorrow-all-may-change."* It made him think of himself as *"a contagious person, a threat or a scourge,"* and he wondered who he might have exposed. Searching his mind, he thought of a number of possibilities, depending on how long he had been carrying the disease; and he wondered where—that is, from whom— he "got it," with an impulse to explain and, possibly, to assign blame. The news, he said, restored a sense of immediacy to his life. He had been distancing himself from AIDS politics in recent months, which, he figured, was related to Nirenberg's antibody-negative report, as well as to his own excellent health and spirits as a result of taking Sinequan. *"I perhaps **did** assume I too was negative. AIDS would hit other people, not me."* That helped to explain, he thought, *"the days & weeks and months"* that he had gone through without paying much thought to AIDS, and the return of his research to his central priority. It helped to explain a lack of attention paid to a friend, Bruce Gowans, who was in the hospital, or to ACT or to the AIDS conference invitation to speak, which he had turned down *"for lack of immediate concerns."* Now he felt the virus in his blood: *"here, now, with the intimacy, the closeness, the marital, no more-than-marital proximity of this serum, this 'immune system' (I is a system?), these heart beats that move the blood around."* He would have to start thinking about and gathering information about the disease again, not so much for himself, he thought, as for others. He would have to have a handle on the necessary information when he told Gail, for instance. *"Just now, I feel mortality has brushed me more forcefully, perhaps even bruised me, with her wing."* The day after writing that passage, Lynch attended another funeral, for Bruce Gowans.

Lynch threw a farewell party for Nirenberg at the end of November but didn't tell his departing lover that he had tested positive. Years later Nirenberg said, "He *never* told me."

On December 2, 1986, the Ontario legislature passed the Human Rights Code amendment, extending protection based on sexual orientation—an important victory, not least because it would provide a means of fighting back against AIDS discrimination. The next day, Nirenberg left for the airport to fly to Vancouver and Lynch headed out to attend yet another funeral, this one for John Hepworth.

In early December he gladly attended a different kind of ceremony—a wedding. George Poland, a former student from St. Michael's College at the University of Toronto, had asked Lynch to be his best man when he married Patricia (Ellie) Perkins in Maryland, on Chesapeake Bay. Years earlier Poland had been a babysitter for Stefan. *"My presence made George happy. He was happy already, effusive with love as I never thought he'd be able to be. I was far less giving, less forthcoming, and seemed to me indeed to be very constricted, and still am, here, now."*

Lynch spent the Christmas holidays in New York, back in the vortex of the epidemic: *"Here the city is brighter than ever . . . except for the waves of the dying. The other day someone mentioned that Mort Gindi was dead—I didn't know he was sick—and Steve Werner is very ill, weak, depleted, skeletal."* There was more. Spiers told him that he had just learned that in Boston Tom Stehling, a former academic who played piano duets with Lynch, was "busting out all over," as Tom himself was putting it, with Kaposi's lesions. Bob Cashman, Ken Calendar's new lover, was also ill, the third partner of Ken's in a row to have AIDS. Bruce Kent (the roommate of another friend, Paul), and Paul himself were also infected. Bruce Schentes and David Cohen were planning to move to Los Angeles. Bruce was convinced that perhaps in the west there would *"be at least a respite for them, time perhaps to deal with Steve's death at last,"* Lynch wrote. *"I say none of these affect me now, perhaps because I'm living past my own death to myself. Bruce says that for him every one is as hard as the 1st, Larry's. He quoted someone else who moved to L.A., 'Promiscuity is over, so I might as well have a kitchen big enough to turn around in.'"*

On December 30, Lewis telephoned Lynch in New York to report that he had a painful case of shingles: *"He was, this morning and this afternoon, on rather heavy narcotics, groggy. But the picture is: he's in pain from the shingles, he's alone, he's very sure now he'd got AIDS, he's scared indeed."* Lynch was ready to return to Toronto, but Lewis told him not to come. Half an hour after his conversation with Lewis, Lynch went off to chair a session on the "Discourse of Homophobia" for the Modern Languages Association. He reminded the audience that for all their academic analysis, homophobia was still present to them "as an immediate and human dilemma." But as he said that, his voice broke, and he was on the verge of tears. All day long he thought of Bill, and only Herb Spiers's admonition to honour Bill's "don't come back tomorrow" kept him from returning the next day, *"to hug him New Year's Eve."*

The MLA session that Lynch chaired had been organized by queer theorist Eve Kosofsky Sedgwick. It was the first time they'd met, but they went on to become close friends. Kosofsky Sedgwick later wrote that Lynch chaired the panel with "amazing dignity and openness" and that the man she met that day was "a Michael made different . . . by the suddenly more graphic proximity of intimate loss—perhaps also by the availability of comfort from friends." She thought he was manifesting an "availability to be identified with and loved."[23]

On New Year's Eve Lynch tallied the dead, the sick, and the (so far) well. During 1986 *"our lives were blessed by growing and by grow-ing loss,"* he wrote. *"Every day a boon, every hour an unexpected gift."*

The end of *TBP,* and important things in life

While Lynch was in New York over the Christmas holidays, *The Body Politic*—the influential "activist academy"—folded. The first week of January Lynch wrote a *"strong & bitter letter to* TBP *collective, angry (now that I learn more details) at their abrupt & selfish dissolution of the paper. I have no trouble seeing that a decision to kill the paper might be wise, or at least necessary, but I'm pissed as vinegar that they did it with-out consulting a wider community."* Lynch was not the only one who was outraged. In a farewell article in *The Body Politic*, Rick Bébout noted that Tim McCaskell was particularly incensed that the decision to close the newsmagazine was "announced to the straight press" before readers, subscribers, volunteers, and contributors were notified. According to Bébout, this was a "slip"—a *Body Politic* press release about its fifteenth anniversary issue brought an inquiry from a local radio station about the publication's future, and the radio station was told the truth. Then the news spread.[24]

In mid-January 1987 Lynch attended the fifteenth anniversary of, and wake for, *The Body Politic*. *"Timmy McCaskell stayed away out of protest against Ken Popert's manipulation of the closing of the paper. I maybe should have,"* Lynch wrote. On reflection he thought that what was lost with the closing of *The Body Politic* was something that had been dead for several years: *"the sense of leading a community in select-ing and shaping the issues, the course of events."* *The Body Politic* had at least been strong for a good long time, he reasoned: *"in touch with what was happening hither and yon (though never enough), cutting at times, politic and impolitic, tense, unresolved, an enemy of blandness, an educator, a difference-maker. How much I learned, **we** learned! But the 'we' I'm speaking of is a 'we' that is no more."*

That "we" included, in his mind, a group who gathered at the communal house on Simpson (*"with Joyce Rock, **the** woman on the collective!"*) to discuss Susan Brownmiller's book *Rape* and whether or not it was anti-gay-male. It included a meeting with John Sewell in his City Hall office just before the first rally around the trial of *TBP*. It included "wrangling" with Ed Jackson or Rick Bébout over a paragraph that was going into the magazine, or with Bill Lewis over an article that the collective was trying to generate. It included the "postpartums" at 435 Roehampton, orchestrated by Lynch, who thought it might be good to host a social gathering away from the office—*"until the potlucks became too mechanical."* It included Lynch's first article, reviewing (*"with a pomposity I'd half unlearn"*) Ian Young, and the Damien struggle, and *"Stefan as a bored little kid playing with paperclips during a collective meeting on Duncan St."* Lynch found himself wishing himself back to those times, thinking, *"with all the poignancy of all the 2:20 a.m. nostalgia a January morning offers, **would we were there again.**"*

Lynch had begun to take tennis lessons in late 1986, hoping to display a new proficiency as a surprise for his tennis-crazed son. Now, during a visit with Stefan and Gail in San Rafael in February 1987, Stefan referred to them as "the tennis family," and that was how Lynch titled a series of "family photos" taken of the three of them at that time. After the photo session, Lynch and his son went into the city and, over burgers at a restaurant, Stefan told his father that in health class the teacher told them to list the ten most important things in their lives—things they could least live without. Next, they had to reduce the list to two things. Stefan said his two things were his father and his mother.

Stefan asked his father what his "two things" would be, and thereafter followed a difficult, complicated conversation. *"I allowed as to how I thought—in these days of so much dying—I could live even w/o him, but I'd find it hard to live w/o accomplishing my book, or w/o generally good health,"* Lynch wrote. Stefan reported that the wife of his teacher hadn't included his teacher in her short list, which Lynch thought might have comforted him about his own choice of things. Most kids apparently listed their parents and friends—people—and Michael suggested that most kids, after all, outlived their parents. Two nights earlier, Lynch said, he had dreamed of having this very same kind of conversation with Stefan, and now here it was taking place right before him: *"the transmission in the dream was that the father/parents teach the child to live on through his/her death."* Stefan asked Michael what his three deepest thoughts were, which caused Lynch to freeze before he finally came out with something about his "current possession" with his book—*"but not my possession by death, not my sense of waste and mediocrity and unaccomplishment.*"[25] Lynch had stopped taking antidepressants at the beginning of the month, and sometimes collapsed into "massive, inexplicable" depressions.

But still, in California he had a sociable and fulfilling time. He gave a talk at the University of California at Berkeley, visited with his friends Bob Reinhard, a former student who had moved to San Francisco, and Allan Bérubé, a gay historian whose partner was dying of AIDS. He pursued friendships with academics Eve Kosofsky Sedgwick and David A. Miller, and was interested to meet with poet Robert Gluck in San Francisco. He was delighted with Stefan and observed: *"We have been happy these three weeks, Gail & Stefan & I, and the surprise is that it's been easy . . . who would ever have thought that Gail & I would mesh so well?"* One night they stayed up until very late talking over their lives, and the deaths in their lives, among other things.

Indeed, Lynch had such a good time that he began to think about looking for a job in California. If Lewis died, he told his diary, there would be no point in staying on at 8 Ross Street or in Toronto.

The fading of the pre-AIDS past

The *"gemstone and lodestone"* of Lynch's return to Toronto in early March was a late Christmas gift from Lewis. It was a beautifully printed and bound copy of "A Week in Nova Scotia"—Lynch's account of a holiday that he and Lewis had taken in 1978.[26] *"Handsome—even with my own misspellings—but most of all a great affectionate gesture from Bill, his strongest ever."*

A couple of days later, Lynch awoke from a dream about his mother and drifted into thinking about the *"pre-AIDS past,"* how it seemed to be slipping further and further away. It had been four years since Larry Okin's death—*"and how many since?"* Lynch was finding as well that the "erotic past" was slipping away too. He fantasized, as he often did, about the pre-AIDS scene, at Fire Island, or in New York, or Toronto, or in a bathhouse—usually imagining a three-way or at least semi-public action, with voyeurs. He found himself slipping into an episode almost forgotten. Some ten years earlier he had gone home with two men from a Columbus Avenue bar. The two men were lovers, and after one of them came they began to fight, and Lynch had to leave. He wrote them a sentimental letter when he got home. *"How far away it all seems! I don't even* **consider** *fucking or getting fucked anymore (though I long for it) . . . I miss The Pines, the bars here, Stages . . ."*

To celebrate Lewis's thirty-seventh birthday, Lynch helped to host a small cocktail party, five days after the actual event, which was March 18. With news coming in of more illness and death—Ken Calendar of the New York "sisters" had Kaposi's sarcoma and Bérubé's partner had died—Lynch's reaction was mainly to celebrate his own health and plan his future. On April 7 he sketched out a schedule for himself through to 1999. According to the plan, he would publish his planned book "Age of Adhesiveness" in 1988 and, in 1991, his Walt Whitman biography.

Lynch travelled to Washington in early April. In a diary entry he described himself at the airport: *"In my gorgeous shirt and leather pants, my white glasses & white tennis shoes, w/black leather shoulder bag, I stand out. Even w/o mousse I stand out. People, not always the ones I'd choose, turn to look . . . Michael Michael you are empowered here, you have privilege here, you are elite—and these do breed indifference, amnesia, unseeing, arrogance."*

Lynch had been interviewed for a CBC-Radio documentary on "AIDS and the Arts" that aired when he was in Washington. The program featured eight gay writers, artists, and critics. Later, when he listened to a tape of the show, he was pleased with the way his reading of one of his poems was introduced—with a background of piano music that established a mood of *"melancholy, haunting introspectiveness."* Although he had not yet told many friends, or even his son, on the radio program Lynch "came out" as having tested HIV-positive: "I am HIV-positive, and a lot of people I know have tested that way and we know very well that tomorrow we could wake up and there's a lesion or something," he said on the nationally broadcast program. "That adds, as one might expect, a little urgency. It also, though, invigorates. I don't know that I've ever felt so invigorated in just day to day life, and the writing comes into that. I edit much more . . . you want what few words that you leave there to matter. It is a great efficiency maker."

Lynch also reflected on AIDS poetry. "We have revived elegy, which was the mode of gay poetry for the last two hundred years." Over the past thirty years or so, he said, elegy had been pushed aside. Writers could say, "I love you" without having to write it to a dead person. Now, Lynch said, he was seeing the "drive to memorialize," again and again. "I think it is an act of memory. We're losing so many people."[27]

Lynch's good friend Ed Jackson was now working at ACT—he began work there as an education officer in 1985—but the diaries of this period make no reference to the activities of the organization that he helped found. In May Lynch had dinner with ACT chair Art Wood, who told *"story after story about his political activism with the big boys (ACT, his link, meets with Chief of Police—whoever),"* but Lynch apparently had no desire to reconnect with the formal world of AIDS. Instead, much of his focus was on writing "Age of Adhesiveness," although he admitted to being *"scared of never finishing it & scared of finishing it."* He decided to ask Bert Hansen, now a history professor at City University, New York, to finish the book if he died before it was completed.

May 4th brought Lynch something to celebrate—a son, Benjamin, was born to his friends George Poland and Ellie Perkins. *"Would you believe, caro libretto, that this sour curmudgeon got excited over a baby today?"* Lynch told his diary. Lynch did not often get the opportunity to celebrate a birth, and he later referred to Benjamin as *"a major change in our lives."* Poland asked Lynch to be Ben's godfather, a responsibility Lynch accepted although he preferred to be known as the infant's *"fairy godmother."*

"AIDS and the Arts" seemed to be becoming a popular topic. In early June a CBC-Television documentary on that subject interviewed Lynch. The program featured him reading his poem "Conspirators."[28] To "illustrate" the poem, the images of various friends who had died were, as their names were mentioned, visually "removed" from a group photo. Introduced as "poet and professor," Lynch told the interviewer: "My poems deal with loss and the kind of anger that comes out of losing so many people where there's still a sense that we just don't need to, or that this is a period in history where we should be able to stop this."[29] Later, Lynch noted wryly in his journal—

*"I'm getting a long ways as an AIDS poet considering that I've hardly published a word! Such is celebrity, I suppose: It's not what you've **done**, it's what a medium says you **are**."*

The 1987 AIDS vigil was held June 11 and Lynch again had trouble with the event, as he had the year before:

> *5 or 6 bland, smarmy, over-homogenized secular (some barely so) pietists. Beating us to death & ennui with their inoffensiveness. The Church of Canada without the Church of Canada. I must simply avoid Jim Bozyk in the future: he can thump his Bible elsewhere. Oh, one speaker of this ilk is o.k., a crumb to the masses, but 6 is deadlier than . . . than Vanna White. Rodney was there, out of the hospital where he went back into (syntax?) yesterday. Graham seems well, beside me . . . Doug Antoski is suicidal, not here (but was at the Diamond Club for "Fashion Cares" last night); Andy Armstrong too weak to leave bed or wheelchair; Barry Covert said his brother Lee is ill & weak; Timmy McCaskell—no AIDS diagnosis I know of, but continued infections—looked peaked. Bill has a bad foot & I feel remarkably healthy & productive, despite a day-long hangover from last night.*

In early July Lewis got a lab result indicating his T-cell count was 140. For a healthy person, a normal result for T-cells, a type of white blood cell involved in the body's immune response, would have been about 800. A decline meant that the body was less able to fight off infection. Still, while doctors kept an eye on T-cell counts, the diagnosis of AIDS depended on the "marker" diseases and infections, like Kaposi's sarcoma and PCP. Lewis was ill, off and on, throughout the summer months of 1987.

For his part, Lynch was often tired and without energy. He had gone back to taking the antidepressant Sinequan, but his sleep remained uneven. He had also been reading about the current patterns of HIV, and that did not help his episodes of depression: *"It's pretty clear now that the only co-factor for the development of AIDS is time. And the viral activity of EBV* [Epstein-Barr virus] *can hardly not be related."* Still, he thought he had no other noticeable weakness, "immunity-wise." But he was assuming that ARC—AIDS-related complex—was at least "very likely" and AIDS "at least likely." He was thinking that he would have to soon talk it all over with Stefan.

Stefan was in Toronto after spending July in France. Though he missed his friends in California, he and his father had a companionable time. Still, Lynch's concern for Stefan was close to the surface. Stefan was fifteen, which was Lynch's age when his father had died. *"I can't help but think of parallels, try to imagine him without me."* When they walked along College Street one night Lynch became lost in those thoughts, and Stefan had to say *"il faut souvire"* twice before his father heard. They tended to keep up a constant talk, about almost everything. And Lynch thought to himself: *"So, let's say Bill dies in 2 years and I a year later. It's summer of 87 now—say I live through the summer of 90, through Stefan's graduation from high school. What do I want to do? What will I leave? Put concretely like this, it's far less a melancholia evoked than a planning plenary."*

On August 13, Lynch bought a copy of the latest *Newsweek*, which featured photographs of three hundred of the several thousand people who had died of AIDS in the past year. He had *"long imagined a yearbook of the dead,"* and now the *Newsweek* layout with its mixed tone and sharp cutlines *"was very yearbookish,"* he wrote. *"I cried, & cried, & cried. Whence this crying? Whence the sense of aptness that comes from the sense of illness or dying? To what degree is this self-pity? Does it accelerate my illness? And is there a way to find the urge to live at the heart of this mournfulness?"* Discouraged and tired, he wrote that he wanted to be "authenticated" as being sick. He had been unwell for some time, off and on, but without a diagnosis. *"I've no interest in anyone these days except Bill and Stefan."*

On his forty-third birthday, Lynch's doctor reported that his T-cell count was 110. *"Very low . . . much lower than I expected though unclear whether it results from HIV activity, the Epstein-Barr situation, or both. Happy birthday Michael—and that's the self-pity of the day."* The only half-decent news concerned the expanded availability of AZT (or zidovudine), which was the first drug approved by the medical establishment to combat AIDS, and had been made available for a limited number of patients in Canada. Lynch would start taking the drug after an upcoming trip to New York City, but did not yet have access to it. *"There's no death sentence yet, but the odds are higher. I may well see 45, but not 50."*

Stefan was still tennis-mad. He played all summer, and he and his father watched and attended matches, including the U.S. Open in New York. *"My image of heaven used to be a disco, but now it's different. Heaven is a tennis court floating, oh, through the sky, where the thunk of balls marks out eons,"* Lynch wrote.

On August 24 Doug Antoski, a professional makeup artist and gay activist, died in his sleep. It was, Lynch wrote, a mercy. *"He was terrified of dying in the horror of John Ward's death, & has tried overdoses at least twice these last few months."* The next day, Ed Jackson and his lover Sam Carvelli had Stefan, Lynch, and Helen Reeves (a fellow tennis fanatic and friend whom Lynch had met through Nirenberg) over for a small dinner to celebrate Lynch's forty-third birthday. Lewis, very ill with a high fever, lack of breath, and near-deafness, was unable to come. Lynch asked his doctor for *"a maintenance dose of Bactrim to fend off PCP until AZT is here, & he said yes."* He also reminded himself to, when in New York, look into getting some aerosolized pentamidine, since *"it isn't here yet."* PCP was the major cause of death for people with AIDS, and aerosolized pentamidine was proving effective in preventing the illness. The problems surrounding the non-availability of aerosolized pentamidine in Canada would soon bring enormous changes to Lynch's life, to Toronto's gay community, and to Canada's medical establishment.

six

THE YELLOW GLOVE

BILL LEWIS WAS admitted to hospital towards the end of August 1987 with PCP—pneumocystis carinii pneumonia—his first bout of the infection. After being been sick for several months, he was relieved to finally have a diagnosis and a treatment plan.

"War on AIDS intensifies on several fronts at U of T" was the headline on an article, featuring Lewis, which had appeared in *The University of Toronto Bulletin* two months earlier.[1] Lewis, by then an associate professor of microbiology with a string of important publications, was profiled because he had just been awarded a $150,000 federal grant to study HIV. His research looked into blood samples collected since 1984 from gay men with swollen lymph glands (often indicators of a weakened immune system) and their healthy partners. The samples had been collected as part of a study conducted by U of T scientists Randy Coates and Colin Soskolne.[2]

Lewis explained in the article that he had tracked the literature about AIDS from the beginning "both because I'm a gay man and because I'm a microbiologist." For a faculty member to so publicly "out" himself as a homosexual was highly unusual. A University of Toronto Homophile Association had been founded in 1969, and a Gay Academic Union in the mid-1970s, but in 1987 only about a half-dozen University of Toronto professors were publicly "out" as homosexuals or lesbians. But Lewis, an otherwise shy and unassuming

121

man, was a dedicated gay activist who had been a member of Gays For Equality in his student days in Winnipeg. He did not, however, tell his interviewer that he was convinced that he was HIV-positive.[3] Nor, apparently, had he told his parents, who were aware of his sexual orientation and supportive.

"We hope that your lab work is going well and that you are making some headway," his father had written to him on July 5. "Your news on the AIDS research is just wonderful, will you be heading up the research? We hope you can find a breakthrough on AIDS as it is causing a lot of trouble and deaths and we think you are more aware of the situation than we are." They were closely following the news and reports about AIDS and hoping that their son's research would help come up with a cure. "We might add that we are very proud of you and the work you are doing and if anyone can solve the AIDS crisis we are betting on you."[4]

Lewis was the first man Lynch had lived with, and among Lynch's many male partners he was the longest lasting and the closest to a peer in age and accomplishments. Lewis had lived at 435 Roehampton Avenue for more than three years, as partner to Lynch and stepfather to Stefan. When Lynch's article "Here Is Adhesiveness" was published in *Victorian Studies*, Lynch dedicated the work "to Bill Lewis, the strength of whose adhesiveness has long excited my own."[5] And when Lewis went into the Toronto General Hospital, Lynch noted in his diary that it was during the same week, ten years earlier, that Bill had moved into Roehampton.

Shortly before Lewis went to hospital, his T-cell count, at 140, was higher than Lynch's, which in late August was 110. Lynch entertained "the possibility of Bill and me dying about the same time," but looking back over the five years of diagnoses and deaths and hopes he concluded, "I really feel that we've years left—and I'll keep operating as if we do!"

On the third of September, Lewis's lung collapsed. He was terrified through the night, and by the time Lynch arrived at the hospital around nine in the morning Lewis was *"a temple of anxiety."* Later a thoracic surgeon installed a drain pipe on his left side, and by around two in the afternoon he was calmer. Lynch was scared—*"not so much during the 'excitement' as after it was over"*—and he imagined himself phoning Gerald Hannon and saying, "We lost him." That night he told his diary, *"That's a phone call I could make,"* but added that he had no intention to do so *"for a long time—25 years or more."*

Lewis's condition continued to worsen over the next few days, and Lynch was haunted by one short line from a poem—"pneumocystis, its velocity." During his hospital stay Lewis scribbled notes from time to time. "I don't think I really want a back rub—disturbs too many painful tubes." "Mostly I just want to be able to see you Gerald, you don't have to do much." "Can I get a little more morphine?"[6]

On Thursday, September 10, Lynch "bit the bullet" and asked friends to come to the Elizabeth Street entrance of the hospital and convene a silent "support circle" on the grass there, in view of Lewis's window. Some thirty-five people showed up at 7 p.m. that evening and formed a circle, holding hands. Sean Kelly, a man from England who was Lewis's lover, was in the room with him, describing what was happening outside. One of the nurses on the floor later told Lynch that in all her career she had never seen such a moving gesture.

It was an extraordinary thing for Lynch to do. Many of those who formed the circle were friends from *The Body Politic* collective, men decidedly more comfortable at protesting and writing political analysis than holding hands in a circle. "We weren't the touchy-feely caretaker types," said Ed Jackson, who was there. "Michael was more likely to cross over to that and set those things up, and so the circle outside Bill's room was both moving and awkward for most of us." Lynch, who would later become the driving force behind establishing Toronto's AIDS Memorial, appeared to easily express both the impulse to action and the impulse to mourn.

On September 16 the medical team told Lewis's parents, Sean Kelly, and Lynch that there was no more hope. The damage to Lewis's lungs could not be reversed. That evening an inner circle—Sean Kelly, Gerald Hannon, Robert Trow, Michael Pearl (a former lover of Lewis's), Randy Coates, Rick Bébout, Robin Hardy, and Stefan—met at 8 Ross. *"I was glad to have them here,"* Lynch wrote that evening. Stefan helped do the "North Carolina thing"—laying out a big spread. Lynch could deal with the rituals, he wrote, but he didn't know how he would be able to deal with Bill's absence from his life: *"the clomp, clomp upstairs, the delight in gardens and cell biology, the shared*

tolerance of each other and shared intolerance of some others. I'll remem-
ber, of course. I told him today these were the happiest years of my life,
here at 8 Ross."

Lewis died at four the next morning. He was thirty-seven years
old. Lynch, devastated, wrote on the front page of his journal: *"Bill to*
hospital 27 August (Thursday). Billy dies 17 Sept—three weeks later
(Thursday). Unbelievable."

While Lynch and Lewis had survived the AIDS deaths of many
friends, particularly U.S. friends, Lewis's was the first death to pene-
trate an inner circle of Toronto activists. The speed of the death took
everyone by surprise. "It remains a mystery," Jackson mused many
years later. Ironically, the Toronto General Hospital was the same
place that had, reportedly, recently begun a treatment for PCP that
was cutting the mortality rate from that infection down from 90 to
10 per cent.[7]

Although they had stopped being lovers years earlier, Lewis had
been one of Lynch's closest friends and familiars. They owned 8
Ross jointly, and most evenings they met to trade news of the day. At
his memorial service, presided over by his friend Robert Wallace,
Lewis was honoured by professional colleagues, including Rose
Sheinin, a biologist and the vice-dean of the School of Graduate
Studies. "Many of us throughout the world are using molecular
genetic concepts and tools developed by Bill. He had an instinct for
where the cutting edge of science would strike gold. Bill was always
ahead of the game," Sheinin said.[8] Harvey Hamburg noted Lewis's
importance back in Winnipeg, in 1974, when Hamburg first came
out and Lewis was one of a small group of gay activists in the city.
Lewis's friend Dr. Dick Smith of Winnipeg, who in 1983 established
the Winnipeg Gay Community Health Centre to do AIDS education,
came to Toronto for the funeral. Lynch, his voice breaking several
times, read "Dirge without Music," a poem by Edna St. Vincent
Millay. The four-stanza poem concludes:

> *Down, down, down into the darkness of the grave*
> *Gently they go, the beautiful, the tender, the kind;*
> *Quietly, they go, the intelligent, the witty, the brave.*
> *I know. But I do not approve. And I am not resigned.*[9]

A couple of weeks after Lewis's death, Lynch was in the audience for "Fruit Cocktail," an annual revue celebrating Toronto's gay community. Afterwards he reflected on his life in Toronto. During the past five to seven years, while he was busy *"doing NYC for the archives, doing the house, doing the deaths,"* Toronto had grown a substantial lesbian and gay community. On October 3 Lynch wrote that when he first arrived in 1971, the only option to participate in a gay community was to be an activist: *"I could act in a smallish group of shit-disturbers, but most of that was action against—I never had a vision of what would come . . . and of course, no one did, history doesn't follow blueprints."* Since that time, a new set of activists had taken the stage. They *"guided and shaped and thought and did, and they brought about the current situation and I did not."* All of this happened, he said, under his nose, and without him fully realizing it.

> *Now here it is, and here (quite solitary) I am. Without Bill, it's me and Othello* [Lewis's cat]. *I don't take help from others easily, and am very prematurely feeling the isolation usually bestowed upon the very old. . . . Perhaps I bury myself in this house as an archives, and become an acquisition to be accessed, a paper or a microform, a historical button.*

The fall and early winter of 1987 would be an understandably difficult period for Lynch. Throughout autumn he addressed his diary to Lewis: *"Billy dear . . . That I'm not emotionally disabled gives pause—shouldn't I be?—yet I know something, from experience, about loss and mourning . . . But how Othello and I miss you."*

A march in Washington

More friends were becoming sick or sicker. At the end of September, Lynch attended a funeral service for thirty-four-year-old Rodney Polich, whom he had met through Sam Nirenberg. Lynch told his diary: For music, *"the choice of Pete Seeger's 'ticky tacky boxes' seemed a bizarre choice given the cheap coffin in front of us. Okay, I'm snobbish in a sense . . . but Rodney deserved better: more Rodney (there certainly were good moments), less family, less chapel."* On November 12 his friend David

Newcome, a patient at Sunnybrook Hospital, was told that he would probably not regain sight in one eye (a month later he was completely blind). The next day, Bob Reinhard called from San Francisco to say he was *"seropositive and scared,"* and a couple of weeks later, Lynch heard that Scott, a San Francisco friend, had just had a bout of PCP.

And Lynch wrote of a "night of panic" in mid-November, when part of him called out for death to come soon: *"Whenever I cry for Billy there's an element of 'why live without him' . . . but there's a strong part saying 'survive, of course' and making plans and looking forward."*

Part of that looking forward had begun on Saturday, October 10, when he left Toronto on an early morning flight to take part in the March on Washington for Lesbian and Gay Rights. It would be a turning point for himself and Toronto gay activists. Washington was *"full of faggots and dykes and even my curmudgeonry won't deter the ebullience of it,"* he wrote. The night before the march featured a "town meeting" on sex and politics—putting the sex back into politics. Lynch noted: *"Assumed and unquestioned = more sex, more good sex, more better sex = a good thing."* He wasn't sure, though, about himself in that equation, at least for now. *"My own libido is on vacation."*

Estimates for the Sunday march, which was organized "for love and for life," ranged from 200,000 (official) to about 600,000. Lynch marched with fellow academics Eve Kosofsky Sedgwick and David A. Miller, and Canadian Robin Hardy, a writer he had known at *The Body Politic*. Hardy had moved to the United States and was writing for *The Village Voice* and other publications. "Among half a million people at the 1987 gay march on Washington, we somehow bumped into each other and spent half a day together," Hardy wrote later. "What was the point of all that work, all that writing?" Lynch asked him. "It'll all be wiped out by AIDS."[10] At the time more than 24,000 people had died of AIDS in the United States; about 1,150 in Canada.[11]

It was during the march that ACT UP, the activist U.S. group founded in New York just seven months earlier, came to nationwide attention within gay and lesbian circles. Lynch's old friend Herb Spiers, a founding member of *The Body Politic*, was by then chair of the powerful issues committee of ACT UP New York, which met regularly at his loft on West 19th Street. "ACT UP was still new; its tactics were still controversial," Spiers recalled. During the March he was with the ACT UP contingent, acting as a sort of monitor. "But I was also free-floating to see what impression the ACT UP contingent was making with the standersby." It was very impressive, he decided. The ACT UP marchers all wore T-shirts emblazoned with the motto "Silence = Death." Lynch and many others wore pins with same slogan.

Two days after the Washington march Lynch joined a civil disobedience demonstration at the U.S. Supreme Court. At issue were two recent rulings—one that denied a woman access to her paralyzed lover and another upholding the criminalization of same-sex sodomy. "Beyond the particulars," wrote Lynch, "these two represented a broad complicity between the courts and other offices of American homophobia—a complicity which continues to increase the epidemic's toll."[12] The march "was a little bit scary, because the police who were responsible for guarding the Supreme Court had a reputation of being harsh," Spiers recalled. Mimicking police, who at earlier AIDS protests had donned rubber gloves, the Supreme Court protestors wore yellow kitchen gloves. Lynch wrote "I love you Bill, 1950–1987" on his yellow glove, and also collected signatures of several fellow protestors, including that of Franklin Kameny, sixty-two, an important early gay leader and founder of the U.S. National Gay Task Force. "Only the two of us over forty recognize Franklin Kameny," Lynch wrote in his poem, "Yellow Kitchen Gloves," about the protest. So (according to the poem) Lynch and a friend, Hank, played "elders," telling other demonstrators about Kameny's past.[13] Lynch was arrested and charged at the demonstration, and spent a brief time in jail. *"The whole weekend energized my spirits out of elegy and into action. I wear sloganned T-shirts again, shouted cheers, even tease myself w/ the idea of starting up an activist AIDS organization here. (God forbid!)"*

Back in Toronto, that's exactly what he did. *"Billy, the activist in me is akickin' and astirrin' again,"* he told his diary (and Lewis) on Oct. 15. *"The city has held up its AIDS budget, and held much of it back from ACT."* The Toronto General Hospital had refused to purchase a PCP nebulizer for the AIDS clinic. *"We must hit the streets . . . The one time in the Washington March rally when I really wept, it was to an old cliché—About our not letting those who've died die in vain. . . . Anger returns, mourn—by organizing."*

Politics and prescriptions

The creation of ACT UP reflected a growing consensus in the gay community that, as writer Randy Shaw put it, "Politely accepting government, scientific, and corporate inaction was equivalent to accepting death sentences for thousands of people potentially infected with or already suffering from AIDS."[14] A key focus for the new organization was the state of AIDS research and the availability of drugs.

On September 10 Lynch had started taking AZT. It was the only available drug that, at the time, was thought to improve the condition of PWAS. The antiviral was not licensed for sale in Canada—indeed, it did not receive a notice of compliance until fall 1990—but had been made available to doctors through a special open-label study in late 1986 and then introduced more widely in 1987. What would prove to be even more important, though, were drugs to prevent the opportunistic infections like PCP, which was the leading cause of death for PWAS. Aerosolized pentamidine was being prescribed by many U.S. AIDS doctors to help prevent the often deadly pneumonia. But it was not available in Canada, and through the fall the issue was becoming part of a new organizing drive. By December 4 Lynch was telling his diary: *"Several phone calls tonight re pentamidine—folks are antsy, maybe will not wait to January for an action—maybe next week?"* A few days later he recorded that a group of ten or eleven of them met at his place for two hours "over hot cider" to form strategy around a possible pentamidine action. *"I was not happy with the meeting but was too tired (and hard of hearing, by the way) to lead,"* Lynch said. Three days later he met with Art Wood, Doug Bonnell, and Phil Shaw from ACT, but noted that *"they must move more slowly on pentamidine."*

In 1986 some U.S. doctors, including those at the Memorial Sloan-Kettering Cancer Center in New York, had begun using pentamidine in an aerosolized form—patients inhaled a mist—to prevent the dangerous pneumonia.[15] In February 1987 researchers recruited by the U.S. National Institute of Allergy and Infectious Diseases (NIAID) to participate in clinical trials rated research into aerosolized pentamidine as a high priority.[16] And by the fall of that year, letters and articles about its use to treat and prevent PCP began appearing in medical journals such as *The Lancet* and *Annals of Internal Medicine*. In Canada, however, pentamidine was only available for intravenous use to treat PCP—not prevent it—and even then it was only available for in-hospital treatment and had to be obtained through Health Canada's Bureau of Human Prescription Drugs.[17]

On November 20 Lynch travelled to New York to get a supply of pentamidine and bought seven doses at $141 (U.S.) each, bringing the tab to nearly $1,000. He investigated and publicized the situation in an article for *Xtra*—"Not My Department: A widely used AIDS drug is kept out of Canada while Ottawa twiddles its thumbs." He discovered that while any doctor in the United States could prescribe pentamidine, now considered by major AIDS doctors to be state of the art therapy for preventing PCP, Canadian officials were waiting for a drug company to propose a drug trial before even considering making it available. It was a clear example of bureaucratic inertia putting people's lives at risk. In an interview with Lynch, the director of clinical trials at the Federal Centre for AIDS, Michael Davis, dismissed the reports about aerosolized pentamidine that had been published in medical journals. "Anyone can get an article in *The Lancet*," Davis told Lynch, "which doesn't prove anything scientifically. People say all sorts of things. It was interesting, but the fact of the matter is it was totally biased . . . one needs a bigger study to prove it." Davis later told *The Toronto Star*, "You can't just say, okay chums, here's the [pentamidine] powder, do what you like. That's stupid. It has to be fully investigated."[18]

For Lynch the question was, who was going "to monitor the slugs in the Health Protection Branch?" Who was going "to pressure the Federal Centre for AIDS to get off its executive ass and work to make aerosolized pentamidine widely and easily available both as treatment and as outpatient prevention?"[19]

A shift in focus

Sharing the pentamidine that he brought back from New York with others—Lynch noted that dosages were packaged so they were most efficiently used by three people at a time—introduced him to other prospective activists who were also ready to organize around the epidemic. *"Scott Cline and one Chuck Grochmal came over to take pentamidine,"* Lynch wrote on December 1. *"I felt like I was running a clinic."* Lynch also shared the aerosolized pentamidine more widely. In December Peter Wood on the Nova Scotia PWA Coalition sent him a cheque for $530 for the drug. "If you know of anyone else who has some for sale, please let us know," Wood wrote.[20]

That autumn long-time gay liberation activist Tim McCaskell had a chance encounter with Lynch at the corner of Beverley and College streets, near where McCaskell was working at the Toronto Board of Education headquarters and not far from Lynch's home. Lynch said he thought Toronto needed something like ACT UP and asked if McCaskell would be interested. McCaskell had "only vaguely" heard of ACT UP, and didn't really have a sense of what it meant, but was interested. McCaskell had been one of the main leaders of the huge demonstration in 1981 after the bathhouse raids, and responsible for international gay news at *The Body Politic*. But he had been less in touch with things since the newsmagazine had folded.

The main source of information for Toronto's gay and lesbian community was now *Xtra*, which had begun life as an ad-heavy supplement to *The Body Politic*. Appearing every two weeks, the tabloid was still ad-heavy and copy weak, but it provided a forum for Lynch's journalism. On November 13, almost two months after Lewis's death, *Xtra* published Lynch's article "Silence Equals Death: US Gays Are Fighting Homophobic AIDS Policies; What about Us?"

The article was, typically, part of a conscious strategy. "When I resumed writing after a silent period," Lynch wrote to a former student in early 1988, "I took on some short journalistic pieces, trying to stir into being a new organization to fight politically for better AIDS policies."[21]

Lynch opened his article by relating a question that a head of a medical science department at the University of Toronto had put to colleagues: "Isn't it the case that, if we just let the epidemic run its course, the homosexuals would die off and, since they don't reproduce, the virus would die off too?" The speaker, wrote Lynch, was a decent intelligent man who would not stick by that scenario if he were under pressure. "But he's not under pressure . . . because gay men in Canada are not putting on pressure where pressure is needed."

Describing his experiences during the March on Washington, Lynch referred to his "twinge of Canadian gay pride" when he had told fellow protestors that Ontario was assuming the costs of his antiviral medication. Some Americans were paying over $10,000 annually for the same medication. Canada had made other advances. The 1969 amendments to the Criminal Code had decriminalized sexual acts between consenting adults, and Ontario's Bill 7, which became law in 1986 and prohibited discrimination on the basis of sexual orientation, had given gays "official legal protections still denied to homos in 49 of the 50 United States." But Ontario gays had not yet come to grips with or monitored other key AIDS issues, including threats to job security, the need for good preventive information, and, of course, treatment. Only when pressure was applied would the established institutions deal with these issues, Lynch argued.

The early years of AIDS in Toronto had been focused on education, prevention, and palliative care. Staff at the AIDS Committee of Toronto struggled to cope with day-to-day issues and funding crises, and they functioned in the midst of waves and waves of deaths. They had little energy to spare for opposing government inaction. As well, government funding and the organization's charitable status limited their ability to protest. Although ACT had finally received some stable funding from the Ontario Liberal government, which came to power in 1985, the organization had charitable status and charities in Canada have to limit political advocacy to a small percentage of their activities. Lynch's new acquaintance Chuck Grochmal put it this way: "ACT is not, regrettably, in the business of social change. For a long time, this was a sticking point with a lot of us who felt they should be."[22] It was much the same in the United States, where the Gay Men's Health Crisis struggled mightily to provide care to the hard-hit New York community.

Hindsight easily points to conditions that bred the emergence of the new activist groups—mounting deaths, government red tape, and inaction—but McCaskell speculated that the course of events might have been different in Canada if Lynch had not spearheaded the formation of the activist group that was taking shape in late

1987. "I think something would have come together, but what would it have looked like?" The strength of the new formation—to be called AIDS Action Now! (AAN!)—came from its combination of experienced activists and new people who, as McCaskell put it, "had been churned up by the epidemic." A key was that Lynch took the initiative when he was still well enough to do so, and he helped to bring together a coalition of people, including McCaskell, George Smith, Gary Kinsman, and some others he was just meeting. The result was a particular history and trajectory. "I think that Michael's initiative there was really crucial in terms of producing that history," McCaskell said.

Seasoned activist that he was, McCaskell recalls that until AAN! was formed, AIDS hadn't struck him as "an issue that politics could be done about." For him, politics was about law, not medicine. The community had experience, especially after the bathhouse raids, with bawdy house laws, and members knew about legal issues surrounding the age of consent and privacy. "Our politics had looked at how the legal system was in fact shaping the lives of gay men," McCaskell said. "But nobody had ever really thought about how the medical system might play a significant role."

There had long been battles over the medicalization of homosexuality. It wasn't until 1973 that the American Psychiatric Association finally removed homosexuality from its official list of psychiatric disorders, the *Diagnostic and Statistical Manual.* For years most of the work around the issue of medicalization centred on psychiatry. To a large degree the delivery of medical services, medical research, the financing or the ethics of medical research, and the role of public health were all new terrain for gay activists. "It is one thing to die, I mean we're all going to have to die," McCaskell said. "But it's another to die when you don't need to." With that experience, with that recognition, comes more questions. "Why don't we need to, what's going on, what could be done differently?" Those questions opened up a whole new area of inquiry or political analysis for the community.

Again, gay activists could take a page from the work of women's health activists, who had already devoted considerable time and thought to the politics of medicine and the health-care system. There was certainly interchange between the two movements. For example, at a later (May 1989) AIDS Action Now! teach-in, Carolyn Egan of the

Ontario Coalition for Abortion Clinics (OCAC) gave a workshop on "How to Attack the State."[23] Another activist, Linda Gardner, was a member of both OCAC and AAN!

Let the meetings begin

During the fall of 1987 Lynch was reading Randy Shilts's *And the Band Played On*, a book widely considered to be an essential history of the early days of the epidemic in the United States: *"I'm halfway through And The Band Played On. Amazed that he can get away with his morality play simplifications, his sheer sleaziness both as a journalist and historian. As always, when faced by a powerful American, I feel useless, helpless and yet determined to kick back somehow."* After he had finished the book, he didn't like it any better: *"stupid shallow, duplicitous and non-historical."* It was a view shared by many AIDS activists, who saw Shilts as glorifying the role of doctors, researchers, and public health officials at the same time as he denigrated the role of gay men and the gay and lesbian community in organizing to deal with AIDS. Lynch had hoped to review Shilts's book for *The Globe and Mail*. He didn't, and instead it received a glowing review from a staff reporter.

But there were other things to do. McCaskell's datebook locates the first official meeting of AAN! at the Carlton Street home of Dr. Michael Hulton on December 20, 1987. Hulton, a British-trained anaesthetist, had immigrated to Canada in 1975, and in the early 1980s he belonged to Gays in Health Care and was an early board member of the AIDS Committee of Toronto. He was so concerned about the treatment of AIDS patients at Women's College Hospital, where he worked, that he cut back on his anaesthesia duties and opened a three-day-a-week general practice for AIDS patients. Frustrated by government policies that limited his ability to provide optimal treatment for his AIDS patients, he was actively lobbying the government to test and release more drugs to combat AIDS-related illnesses.

Around the same time action was taking place among a network of Toronto doctors who were establishing the HIV Primary-Care Physicians Group. Dr. Wayne Boone initiated the network so that front-line doctors could share knowledge and contacts. At the time, members of the Toronto network had a combined load of 1,600 patients who were infected with HIV.[24]

McCaskell recalls fierce debate during those early meetings about the nature of the proposed activist organization. It took time to determine how the new organization would be shaped. At an early meeting, one participant with strong opinions, Alan Dewar, fairly shouted out, "This has got to be a *gay* organization. If it isn't I'm not interested in having anything to do with it." Dewar believed that ACT and other organizations like the People With AIDS Foundation had often downplayed gayness in order to gain more respectability with funding organizations—part of a not rocking the boat attitude.[25]

While all of this was going on, Lynch—still teaching full-time and mourning Lewis's death—found time to keep up the pressure through his journalism. Near the end of December, *Xtra* published "Killing Us Softly," an article about Toronto city alderman Tony O'Donohue, who had consistently tried to block the city Public Health Department's attempts to produce accurate information about safer sex. In his campaign O'Donohue had enlisted as allies the likes of Cardinal Carter of the Roman Catholic Church and Mayor Art Eggleton.[26] At issue this time was a pamphlet about the correct use of condoms.

Lynch's article also criticized ads about AIDS in Toronto's transit system. The posters advised people to "Choose to be faithful"—advice that was, to be sure, neither specific nor necessarily protective. Instead Lynch argued that two of the classic phrases of safer sex education—"NO CUM IN BUM" and "ON ME, NOT IN ME"—should be in brochures, posted in bus shelters and on other public transit locations, and provided to school AIDS programs. The piece was an echo of his earlier argument, made in *The Body Politic* in January 1986, for using explicit language to promote safer sex among gay men.[27]

As 1988 began, though, Lynch was turning his attention full force in another direction: to treatment activism—to a critique of biomedical research and government regulatory procedures.

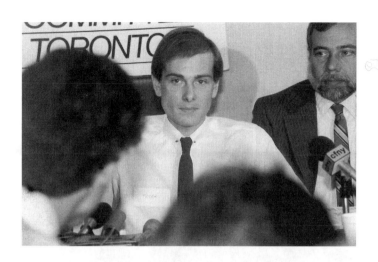

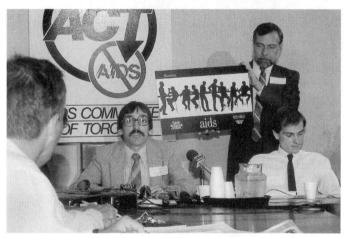

TOP: *Peter Evans at the July 19, 1983, press conference announcing the existence of the* AIDS *Committee of Toronto (*ACT*). Evans, a stage designer, was the first Canadian with* AIDS *to "go public"—to allow himself to be photographed and quoted. He died on January 7, 1984.* (Photo: Debra Bloomfield)

BOTTOM: *Bill Mindell (seated on left), Bert Hansen (standing), and Peter Evans. At the press conference announcing* ACT*, the Toronto Public Health Department unveiled the "Numbers" poster that it had developed in conjunction with* AIDS *activists. The message of the poster—showing silhouettes of men at a bar—was reduce risk by reducing the number of sexual partners.* (Photo: Debra Bloomfield)

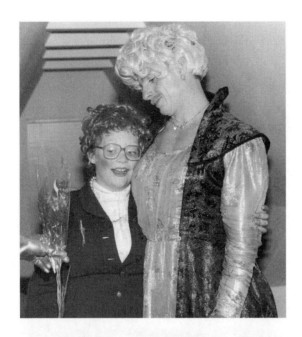

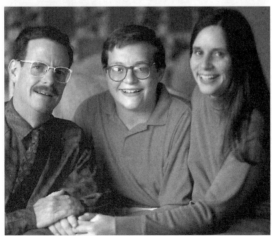

Top: *Stefan and Michael Lynch at a Hallowe'en party, 8 Ross Street, Oct. 29, 1983. Stefan, eleven, wore a red suit that had belonged to his grandmother Lynch and "looked like a classic librarian." One partygoer, worried about their future "mental health," asked Stefan and his two friends (also in drag) why they didn't dress up as, for example, baseball players. "It's easy," Stefan replied. "That wasn't the theme of the party." (From Lynch's diary.)*

Bottom: *Michael, Stefan, and Gail Lynch, February 1987, in San Rafael, California. Lynch dubbed this photo "the tennis family." He began taking tennis lessons in 1986 to surprise and impress his tennis-mad teenage son.* (Photo: Peggie McOmie)

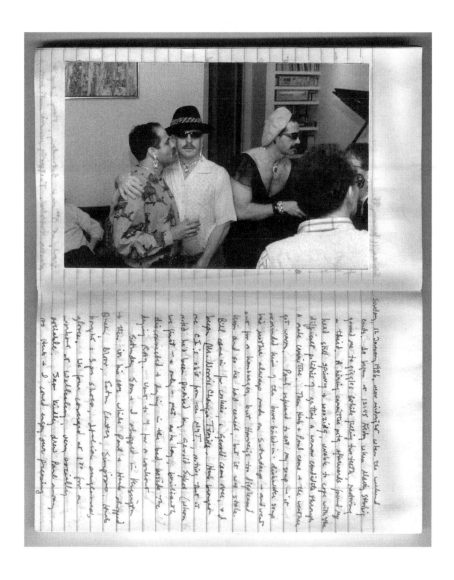

This page is from diary no. 50 of Michael Lynch's set of sixty-five diaries. The photo, which appears opposite an entry for Jan. 12, 1986, was taken at a party at 8 Ross Street, with Sam Nirenberg and Michael Lynch (embracing) and Herb Spiers. Visiting from New York, Spiers "garbed himself in a series of garbs, each with an entrance AND exit," Lynch wrote in his diary (courtesy of CLGA).

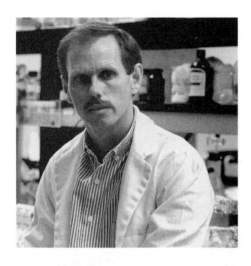

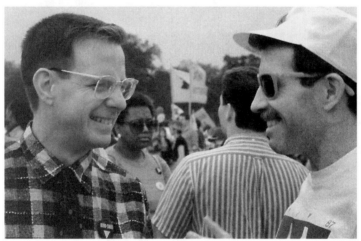

Top: *Bill Lewis, associate professor of microbiology, in his University of Toronto lab. Lynch wrote "I LOVE YOU BILL" on the yellow glove that he wore at the 1987 U.S. Supreme Court protest.* (Photo: Steve Behal)

Bottom: *Lynch (left) with fellow academic David A. Miller at the March on Washington for Lesbian and Gay Rights, Oct. 11, 1987.* (Photo: Eve Kosofsky Sedgwick)

seven

FROM ELEGY TO ACTION

IT WAS JUST BEGINNING to get light outside when Lynch roused himself for a 7:15 a.m. interview with the local CBC-Radio morning show. Later that day—Tuesday, January 26, 1988—he wrote in his diary: *"'And now,' said the lead-in, 'AIDS Action Now!' 1st time I heard the new organization name over the air."*

In the following five months the activist group would get off to a dynamic start. Experienced political activists together with new recruits harnessed the grief, frustration, and anger of years of AIDS losses and government neglect into action on behalf of those already infected. Hundreds of supporters would attend an inaugural public meeting, and soon thereafter the organization would stage a series of well-organized and effective public protests in Toronto and Ottawa.

But when Lynch did that first radio interview, AIDS Action Now! was not yet a full-fledged reality. A small group of activists had been meeting for several months, and Lynch himself had written a number of articles, several published in *Xtra* and one in *The Globe and Mail*, which identified key issues that drove the formation of the new group. His most recent article, "Nothing Doing—Ottawa and AIDS: Spend almost nothing, do almost nothing, take all the credit," took the form of an open letter to federal Health Minister Jake Epp and appeared in *Xtra* on January 15. The Federal Centre for AIDS had, Lynch argued, done nothing to "really address the two crying needs

139

for federal AIDS leadership: explicit education for those who are not infected with HIV and aggressive development of drugs to treat those already infected."

So the groundwork had been laid for an organization, and Lynch's early-morning radio interview served as an advance notice for AAN!'s first press conference, to be held a few hours later. But there had not yet been any public meetings or attempts to garner wide support.

Lynch was himself coping with HIV-related health problems, even as he was teaching a full course load at the University of Toronto, writing articles, and attending meetings. He had been taking AZT since September 1987, and undergoing occasional blood transfusions to combat the anaemia that was a common side effect of the antiviral drug. He was also regularly inhaling the aerosolized pentamidine he had brought in from the United States to prevent PCP, and was being treated by a practitioner of Chinese traditional medicine recommended by Tim McCaskell.

The day before his radio interview, Lynch had chaired a four-hour meeting aimed mainly at planning an upcoming community meeting. *"Thank God for George Smith, Timmy McCaskell, Art Wood and other Tired Old Activists—and for the relatively new minds and bodies,"* he wrote in his diary. *"We TOAs can trust each other, or at least know how far to trust each other, and the newer blood brings help. I feel an ease in this that's so different from the Damien Committee days, and from the early days of ACT. Is there a luminosity that comes with a sense of mortal limits? Perhaps . . . but surely the main factor here is experience, shared communal experience."* The experience of past activism would come into play when AAN! drafted a constitution the following April. It was based on two other constitutions—that of the Right to Privacy Committee, which emerged following the police raids on the bathhouses of the late 1970s and early 1980s, and of the Canadian Committee against Customs Censorship, established in 1986 to fight the officialdom that targeted and censored gay and lesbian material entering the country.[1]

The formation of AAN! soon brought academic Gary Kinsman back to Toronto AIDS activism. After working at ACT for six months in its earliest days, Kinsman had spent the intervening years at universities studying and teaching, and he had authored one of the key works in Canadian gay studies, *The Regulation of Desire*, a history of sexuality in Canada. In his view, AAN!'s origins rested in three groups: seasoned gay activists living with HIV, like Lynch, Smith, and McCaskell; HIV-negative gay activists like himself; and primary-care doctors concerned about access to drugs and treatment, like Michael Hulton, Denis Conway, Wayne Boone, and Philip Berger.

Smith, who had chaired the Right to Privacy Committee, was a sociologist teaching at the Ontario Institute for Studies in Education. Kinsman later credited Smith for insisting that the name of the new organization should be a slogan. According to McCaskell, Smith was "really the intellectual power behind the organization and the strategies we used—organizing a large public meeting, getting personal stories from the community about what was wrong, and beginning to channel the anger and energy into an actual political force."

But AAN! also brought in new people. Among them was Alan Dewar, who had been an alderman for the city of Oshawa and a senior civil servant for the Ontario government. Lynch had written about this "Alan" in an opinion piece published in *The Globe and Mail* in December 1987. At the time, Dewar had already been hospitalized twice with PCP; he could not tolerate standard treatments and had no access to aerosolized pentamidine. Dewar, said McCaskell, "had played by the rules all his life." Now, suddenly, "he realized he was a dying disposable queer, and he was enraged, and part of that was his white male privilege suddenly being stripped from him. His life was coming to a close and he knew it, and the stuff he had believed in terms of a good conservative state was not delivering."

AAN!'s strength, as it developed, was its ability to bring together people of different political persuasions to focus on the immediate issues facing people with AIDS. The organizers deliberated long and hard to determine just what the organization's basis of unity should be. As McCaskell put it, the members of AAN! did not necessarily have to agree "on national liberation in Mozambique or who was more oppressed, women or Black folk, or any of those questions that plagued the left" during the previous decade or so. What they were doing was pulling together a coalition or alliance of people from a wide variety of different backgrounds. Still, the vast majority of those affected by AIDS in Canada were gay men.

Treatment activism in Vancouver

While AAN! emerged as the foremost activist group in Canada, it was in Vancouver, where the provincial Social Credit government had been particularly unresponsive to the concerns of people with HIV/AIDS, that treatment activism first emerged. In the early years of the epidemic, British Columbia had the highest number of cases per one million population in the country. As of February 1987 the province had sixty cases per million, compared to twenty-four in Ontario and twenty-five in Quebec.[2]

In 1985 Kevin Brown, a PWA and former teacher, had a personal meeting with Dr. A.J. (Bert) Liston, assistant deputy minister of the federal government's Health Protection Branch (HPB) in the Health and Welfare Department. Brown realized that government experts had no handle on AIDS—that "It was just beyond them." Liston told Brown that experimental AIDS drugs would be released on "compassionate grounds," but when Brown's doctors applied for the drugs, they were turned down. Brown's doctor, Hilary Wass, a hematologist, shot back that the HPB was failing to fulfil its mandate, which was to administer to the health needs of all Canadians, and that included PWAS. "The whole thing suffers from a lack of direction and a lack of centralized organization. If there was an epidemic of smallpox, can you imagine the resources that would be mobilized to fight it?" Wass asked.

Brown himself would later acknowledge his trepidation about speaking out about AIDS: "When I first went public, I thought I'd walk the streets the next day and be clubbed like a Harp seal." But he did speak out, telling interviewer Laurier LaPierre in 1986 that he believed he should have the chance to explore every opportunity to save his life. "I'm finding the Canadian government has denied me that opportunity. I feel very much led down the garden path—my doctors were misled by the government on several occasions."[3]

Instead of waiting for government approval of experimental drugs, Brown began trying to prolong his life by obtaining a personal supply of Ribavirin (an antiviral) and Isoprinosine (an immune modulator) from Mexico. In 1986, with Warren Jensen and Taavi Nurmela, he founded the Vancouver Persons with AIDS Coalition for people with

HIV/AIDS. "A lot of organizations have more of a palliative approach. . . . We want to make it harder for you to die," Nurmela explained in a panel discussion in 1986.[4]

That year the World's Fair Expo 86 was attracting thousands of visitors to the city, and volunteers from the newly formed coalition headed out to the streets to solicit signatures for a petition demanding that experimental AIDS drugs be released on compassionate grounds. At the time, one of the Catch 22s facing B.C. patients was that if AIDS patients ever did manage to get drugs released on compassionate grounds, they could not take them because there was no viral laboratory in British Columbia that allowed doctors to monitor blood samples. Indeed, the first AIDS protest in Canada, held March 26, 1986, on the steps of the legislature in Victoria, B.C., was staged by the Vancouver Persons with AIDS Coalition to demand a viral laboratory in the province. Even when a laboratory did finally open in 1987, after protests by activists and lobbying by Pat Carney, federal MP for Vancouver Centre, its existence still did not lead to the release of experimental drugs.

In June 1986, PWA coalition members Brown and Warren Jensen travelled to Ottawa. Armed with a petition signed by close to six thousand people, they met with Health Minister Epp. "I'm tired of going to funerals," Brown said."I'm tired of burying my friends."[5]

Michael Davis, head of the infection and immunology division of the Health Protection Branch, countered that there were no effective drugs to combat AIDS, that the Branch was trying to get as many "drugs with potential" out as it could. At the time only two drugs— Cyclosporine, an anti-rejection drug used by transplant patients, and Suramin—had been approved for clinical trials in Canada. The trial of Suramin never did begin, because U.S. data suggested horrific toxicity. Cyclosporine also proved not to be helpful.[6] Davis argued that if the government handed out drugs not proved to be effective, researchers and manufacturers would prematurely abandon further studies of drugs. He said he had to balance the needs of patients dying today of AIDS against the projected needs of thousands of Canadians expected to die of the disease in the future. But as Brown said later: "We're dealing with a life and death issue here. If we wait for something to be proven, it may be too late. I may not be alive, and I want my chance now."[7]

Activists argued that some experimental drugs could be released on compassionate grounds, that individuals should be able at least to try to use them. They also argued the need for more drug trials. They complained that the federal government was insensitive to the needs of AIDS patients. "They call it cautious," Jensen said. "They're looking at saving money instead of saving lives. We're not saying they should allow our doctors to run loose with drugs; but [at least] they should permit our doctors to administer similar drug trials (to those) being conducted in the USA and Europe."[8]

Brown and Jensen had probably seen AIDS Treatment News, a U.S. newsletter started up in 1986 by John S. James. That year's September issue, "What's Wrong with AIDS Treatment Research," surveyed the meagre research landscape. James concluded with a rallying cry and an observation:

> But no longer can we rely entirely on government-sponsored organizations or on the medical-industrial complex for our understanding of what is happening with treatment research and development. . . . The companies who want their profits, the bureaucrats who want their turf, and the doctors who want to avoid making waves have all been at the table. The persons with AIDS who want their lives must be there too.[9]

In November 1986 the Canadian government decided to release AZT to a limited number of patients under what Dr. Norbert Gilmore, chair of the National Advisory Council on AIDS, called an "open label compassionate access program." Some two months earlier a Phase II clinical trial of AZT in the United States had been ended early because the drug was deemed effective—patients had shown some clinical improvement—and it was considered unethical to continue to give a placebo to the control group of patients in the double blind trial.[10] Under the Canadian scheme, AZT was to be released only to doctors or pharmacists for use by patients who had already had PCP. And since the government needed to collect data to justify the release of the drug, Gilmore himself composed and typed up a form to be sent to pharmacists.

Kevin Brown did finally gain access to AZT on December 3, 1986. Unfortunately, the drug would prove—especially at the early high dosages—toxic for many people. The troubles of PWAS in Vancouver continued on for some time; and until 1989 AZT would be the only AIDS drug available in Canada. In 1987, after B.C. health minister Peter Dueck refused funding to AIDS Vancouver, he told a television audience that the organization could "help their own." Dueck later said his remarks were not a slur, and proceeded to compare PWAS to groups like Alcoholics Anonymous or "a society formed to look after mentally handicapped."[11]

AAN! holds its first press conference

"If this syndrome were affecting 1,500 Canadian Boy Scouts, neither Mr. Epp nor Ms. Caplan would be reacting with such armchair leisure," Lynch told the January 26, 1988, press conference that announced the formation of AAN! At the time 1,500 Canadians had been diagnosed with AIDS, and Lynch was putting federal health minister Epp and provincial health minister Elinor Caplan on the hook. "They are moving too damn slow. They are letting us die off because we are gay."[12]

Lynch lambasted Epp and the Health Protection Branch, which, he noted, had made AZT available only after organized pressure from the gay community. "We find no indication that either the HPB or the Federal Centre for AIDS has undertaken ANY proactive search for promising drug trials."

Other speakers at the press conference included Art Wood, chair of ACT, John Hamilton, chair of the People with AIDS Foundation (established in 1986), and Dr. Wayne Boone, a family physician and co-chair of the HIV Primary-Care Physicians Group. Boone outlined "large deficits" in the delivery of health care, including uncoordinated care and inadequate policy and procedures to allow patients access to experimental drugs. The provincial advisory body on AIDS had made no attempt to share information with general practitioners, he said. Because only specialists could prescribe AZT for AIDS patients, there had been delays of up to six weeks for patients who qualified for the open trial, but had to wait to see a specialist.

On January 29, Toronto's largest free-distribution weekly tabloid, *NOW*, published a feature on AAN!: "Advocacy Action on AIDS: Like no other patients before them, people with AIDS are organizing against a cumbersome health system to prolong their own lives." Lynch wrote in his diary: *"I'm astonished at our power to **have** a powerful group just by virtue of **saying** there's one. Premature substantiation?"* He thought back to "the old days" of the Coalition for Gay Rights in Ontario and the Damien crisis—*"We **were** a group and the media never took note."* Lynch had chaired the defence committee for John Damien—the jockey fired because of his homosexuality—who had become a cause célèbre of the gay community, but in this reflection Lynch seemed, perhaps naively, to be ignoring a huge difference between the two events—namely, media appeal. AIDS, for mainstream journalism, was a far bigger story. In 1988 AIDS deaths were mounting in Canada, and the epidemic had become big, and continuing, news. *The Toronto Star* had a full-time AIDS reporter, and *The Globe and Mail* was also following the issues. TV news broadcasts offered regular and special coverage. Lynch himself had been interviewed by various media outlets. At one point he even referred to himself in his diary as a "media slut."

Indeed, Lynch was gaining something of a public profile. On *The Journal* (CBC-TV) in early January, he talked publicly about having AIDS in order to bring attention to AIDS issues, including the reality that some PWAS were facing job loss because of their diagnosis. The appearance prompted an admiring letter from a political scientist at the University of Alberta. The academic wrote, "It is very rare that an individual uses the security of a tenured academic position to accomplish some public good, at the risk of some backlash against them personally. I want to commend you for your honesty and courage." Lynch wrote back, thanking the academic for a "very welcome" letter. But he added: "I must disagree with you on the issue of honesty and courage. Tenure actually *lessens* the need for these things! I risked very little. What's so appalling is that the tenure system seems to select 'in' those who are least willing to use the decent security it offers."[13]

The *NOW* article contained another bit of news: the federal government had okayed a trial of aerosolized pentamidine, although no formal agreement had been signed. "There is far too much optimism about the drug," Michael Davis, now director of clinical trials for the Federal Centre for AIDS, told the tabloid. "It may have a place, but it's not the magic treatment that people make it out to be."

Davis might have thought aerosolized pentamidine was over-rated, but Anthony Fauci, head of the U.S. National Institute of Allergy and Infectious Diseases, had a different understanding of its merits. A few months later, in April 1988, when Fauci had to testify under oath before a congressional committee, he told the committee that if he had AIDS and had already had a bout of PCP, he would obtain and use aerosolized pentamidine.[14] It was a shocking admission from a man who hadn't managed, thirteen months after aerosolized pentamidine was considered a high priority for testing, to even launch a trial of the drug. But it did show considerably more awareness than Canada's bureaucrats.

The community meeting and fractured services: the stigma continues

The core group for AAN! decided to launch the organization with a community meeting at Jarvis Collegiate Institute. The location was an obvious choice. Large public meetings at Jarvis, Toronto's oldest high school, had been strategically used to organize resistance after the 1981 police raids on the bathhouses and to launch the AIDS Committee of Toronto.

Glen Brown arrived in town from Regina, where he had been working on *Briarpatch* magazine and dreaming of Toronto. For a budding community activist and leftist, and gay kid, in Regina, *The Body Politic* had been his "rock." It made him realize that he was not alone, that there was "something more than just a bunch of people, there was a community and a politicized community." He had, he said, been "able to read Tim McCaskell talking about the links between international solidarity and lesbian and gay stuff and Michael Lynch talking about sexual liberation, not just civil rights." He had seen articles about the AIDS epidemic that were not just medical but political.

Brown said he was attracted to AAN! flyers and posters that promoted the Jarvis meeting. "TOO DAMN SLOW! Our friends are dying while bureaucrats fiddle," screamed the posters, which featured a line drawing of a caveman/Thor-type figure holding a hammer, the "Silence = Death" slogan from ACT UP, and the tag line "AIDS Action Now!" The design was by Graham (Gram) Campbell, a graphic artist and the partner of archivist Alan Miller.

About four hundred people showed up to that first AAN! meeting, on February 4. Glen Brown went, not knowing many people in town, and there before him, at the front of the room, he said, were "these incredibly powerful speakers . . . names that I knew as heroes from reading *BP*. Tim McCaskell, Michael Lynch, very passionate and eloquent, Gary Kinsman." He had already read Kinsman's book, *The Regulation of Desire*. "I'd never heard of Chuck Grochmal before that evening and all of a sudden here is this guy saying things in a really straightforward way, and it was hard not to be mobilized, not to be moved."

From April 1988 until his death in 1990, Grochmal would write a regular column in *Xtra*, lucidly and wryly commenting on key political and personal issues relating to living with HIV/AIDS. That night Grochmal illustrated the need for an AIDS treatment centre in Toronto by holding up a fistful of plastic hospital identity cards, noting that he was being treated in at least five separate hospitals because they had divided up patient care. "I spend about a week every month running around from institution to institution," he told the crowd. "AIDS isn't the only thing that's making me feel like shit . . . I'm exhausted just running around."[15]

Other cities, such as Vancouver and San Francisco, had decided to centralize AIDS care in one hospital so that the facility could build up expertise in treatment. In Toronto the medical authorities had decided that centralizing care would scare off other patients, Dr. Michael Hulton later explained. "So each hospital went through a learning experience and patients suffered"[16] In fact, he commented, turf wars between hospitals and key AIDS specialists probably contributed more to the diffusion of AIDS care in Toronto than concern about "scaring off" patients.

Dewar told the gathering about his experience with the standard treatment for PCP, Septra (also known as Bactrim), a drug used to treat patients with immune suppression. Septra was first used with AIDS patients recovering from PCP in the early 1980s, but was toxic for many of them.

After Dewar found out he couldn't tolerate Septra or the other standard treatment, intravenous pentamidine, his immunologist told him aerosolized pentamidine was less toxic. But the drug wasn't available in Canada, so Dewar was going to Buffalo to get it. "I can afford it, but not all of us have the money or the strength. Why is this not seen as intolerable treatment?" Dr. Hulton had a California medical licence (in addition to his Canadian papers) and could write prescriptions for aerosolized pentamidine to be filled at a Buffalo drug store. He later discovered that Ontario licensed doctors could also write prescriptions that could be filled in Buffalo; hence the emergence of the Buffalo connection.[17]

The Jarvis meeting also heard testimonials from the audience, including one nurse who said he discovered doctors "had placed his dying friend on the 'do not resuscitate' list without consulting him or anyone connected to him."

AIDS was an unusual affliction because it consisted of a set of different diseases, George Smith explained. The illness, presumably the HIV (human immunodeficiency virus), depressed the immune system, making people vulnerable to opportunistic infections and conditions. When people contracted those so-called "defining" illnesses—including PCP, toxoplasmosis, cryptosporidiosis, and Kaposi's sarcoma—they were deemed to have AIDS. Yet there was no standard of care, no comprehensive plan for care, and "no real commitment on the whole to deal with AIDS." Medical specialists did not feel obligated to see patients. Looming restraints on health-care spending made activism essential. "If we're not in there fighting, we'll be pushed to the back of the line," Smith said. And the AIDS struggle was not just in the interests of the gay community, he argued. "We fight for the IV drug users, for the babies born with AIDS, for the hemophiliacs and for the Third World, where HIV infection is rampant."

After the speeches, audience members—mostly white and gay men—went off to different rooms in the high school to join the various subcommittees, including fundraising, media, and public action. When the whole group came back together the participants endorsed four demands: 1) trials of aerosolized pentamidine should be instituted across Canada; 2) the Federal Centre for AIDS should seek out new drugs and promote their testing; 3) Health and Welfare Canada should credit drug tests done in other countries; and 4) the Ontario Ministry of Health should provide co-ordinated care for PWAS.

"Dear Billy, I get rather weak and shivery addressing this one to you," Lynch wrote in his diary on Feb. 4. *"We had the community meeting for AIDS Action Now! tonight . . . It went very smoothly: rather laid back, but with no shortage of speakers from the floor and no contesting of key issues or directions. The energy level was not like after the bath raids, with anger on the cuff, but seemed submerged, afraid perhaps to burst out."* Someone at the meeting had said to Lynch, "All we can do is cry." To which he replied, "I've cried enough—no more." A good many people had come up and thanked him for his activism—enough, he wrote, *"to make me feel recognized, loved, appreciated, and I'm glad. Still, it seems to come in conjunction with the syndrome, as part of a long swansong ahead. I used to want the big obituary, now I want the big life: long and effective."*

As Grochmal told the meeting, hospital services for PWAS were fractured; and outside of hospitals, not that many family doctors or specialists were able and willing to treat AIDS patients. "Doctor dumping"—when a doctor unceremoniously decided to no longer treat someone who tested HIV-positive—was not uncommon. The network of general practitioners who were treating the bulk of AIDS patients was overburdened, and some doctors who did treat PWAS knew very little about the syndrome. AIDS was a relatively new syndrome (physicians had to scramble to keep current), and it manifested itself in a range of illnesses and symptoms that took time and patience to diagnose and attempt to treat. Under Ontario's predominant fee-for-service payment system, longer appointments meant less income for doctors.

It was around this time that Darien Taylor had a run-in with a Hamilton, Ontario, doctor. Taylor had tested positive in 1987 when she was teaching in a remote area of Zimbabwe, and when she returned to Canada the doctor told her that she should *spray her toilet seat with Lysol after every use.* "It was ridiculous," she said, but it clearly conveyed to her that she was "this fearsome infectious body that can infect people in many ways, all the time. It was rubbish then and it is rubbish now. But that is the mythology—that people with AIDS are unpredictably infectious. I think that drives the stigma and the fear."[18]

As Taylor's story shows, the medical profession was not innocent of ignorant fear-mongering around AIDS. Even though it was already clear that HIV was actually very difficult to transmit, some hospital nurses persisted in entering the hospital rooms of people with AIDS covered up in "space suits," a practice that persisted in some Canadian hospitals well into the 1990s.

The stigma surrounding AIDS was pervasive, and the persistence of some ugly hospital experiences was part of the driving force behind the setting up of Casey House, a free-standing hospice exclusively for people with AIDS. The hospice opened in March 1988, located in a large, beautifully renovated house on Isabella Street, just a few blocks from Church and Wellesley. It was the first free-standing hospice in Canada. But there was no overlap between AAN! members and those who toiled to establish Casey House. Chiropractor Bill Berinati, a friend of Lynch's, was on the board of Casey House and would occasionally regale Lynch with tales of Casey House politics, but that was the extent of the crossover. The exclusive focus of AAN! was the treatment needs of people with AIDS. The goal of Casey House was to provide better deaths.

This difference prompted Lynch, in 1990, to write a scathing letter to *Toronto Life* magazine, which had published an excerpt from a book about Casey House:

> Patrick Conlon's paean to Casey House ("Coming Home," May 1990) fails to situate its opulence with respect to other issues in HIV care. As a Person Living With AIDS I welcome Casey House, and hope that if the need arises I'll be one of the lucky thirteen whom the gods grant beds there. A nurse for every two and a half patients? All those smart Italian furnishings? Who wouldn't want to die there? But its smart extravagant success in fundraising raises a bothersome issue for those of us trying to live with AIDS: is

Toronto's philanthropic community more eager to fund our dying than to fund our living?[19]

Social service vs. political activism

Torontonians had, at Glad Day and other bookstores, ready access to U.S. gay publications covering AIDS politics south of the border. But the success of AAN! hinged in part on the information that some members, like Lynch, gleaned first-hand about activism during trips to the United States. In New York, playwright Larry Kramer spear-headed the need for an activist organization by lambasting Gay Men's Health Crisis, the service organization that he had helped to found in 1981. In "An Open Letter to Richard Dunne and Gay Men's Health Crisis," published in the January 1987 New York Native, Kramer berated Dunne for complicity with the status quo. "You have become simply another city social services agency," he declared. Kramer went on to ask a series of questions. "Why have you not been in the fore-front of demanding the immediate availability of drugs on a 'compassionate usages' basis to those who are in the throes of dying anyway?" and "Why do you not ride herd on Research?" and "What has happened to your presence in Washington?" Kramer continued, "There is noth-ing in this whole AIDS mess that is not political! How can you continue to deny this fact and assert that your role must remain unpolitical?"[20]

Given his regular visits to New York and friendship with Herb Spiers, who was chair of ACT UP's issues committee, Lynch was famil-iar with the hostile and antagonistic climate that had developed there and was determined that the same experience should not happen in Toronto. In New York, Tim McCaskell pointed out, Gay Men's Health Crisis, which was the original social service organization, and ACT UP were "like dogs and cats, at each other's throats." In Toronto, said Ed Jackson, who worked with ACT at the time, "Michael never tried the Larry Kramer approach—you know, ACT is a failure, get rid of it, we need something else." Lynch was always very careful to keep people at ACT informed about what AAN! was up to, and indeed ACT's board chair Art Wood was in on the formation of AAN! Lynch "stressed the need for an organization without the responsibility and ties—the strings that came with government funding—to do its work," Jackson said. The idea was that the group would really be able to pressure the government and medical institutions, to get things done, to engage in radical agitation, organize demonstrations. "ACT UP and AAN! kind of pooled some of the anger that wasn't addressed by simply setting up service organizations that did education and support." According to Jackson, what happened in New York was "the usual sort of thing of looking for the enemies amongst you, turning on your friends to pick on because they are easier to fire at than the enemies who are elsewhere."

For McCaskell, the New York experience, which he attributed to "American nastiness," provided an object lesson for the Toronto group. The Toronto group made a conscious decision early on to be different, to recognize the two different needs: social services for people who are sick and dying; and an organization that could be more outspoken, that could charge ahead on issues for the community. The group recognized that organizations dependent on government funding could not be political in the same way because of legal restrictions—Canadian charitable organizations, by law, can devote only a very small part of their activities to "advocacy."

"Many people were pissed off at ACT because they hadn't been more outspoken in terms of politics, and what we said was, look, we need another organization to do that, that isn't ACT's job," McCaskell recalled. "We need a division of labour, because you can't expect a service organization to do that kind of work." The core of people with political experience going back to the bath raids was able to jump in and point out that the Toronto organizations should be allies, that they should co-operate whenever they could, and not bad-mouth each other when they couldn't find common ground.

Indeed, two days after the Jarvis meeting Lynch wrote a glowing article for *Xtra* about Joan Anderson, outgoing chair of the board of ACT, and Art Wood, her successor. Anderson, he wrote, brought internal and financial stability to an organization that had been in rough shape when she became chair in 1986. Wood, meanwhile, pledged to establish "advocacy leadership."[21] Lynch said he wrote the piece because he liked them both, shared their commitment, and admired their accomplishments. He knew *"that even a little piece like this,*

*wrapping fish next week, will make some small difference for ACT—
encourage the staff, reassure the milder doubters.*" It was a heartfelt, but
also a strategic, homage. Despite his critique of educational cam-
paigns aimed at the "general public," Lynch believed that the AIDS
Committee of Toronto, with Ed Jackson, Rick Bébout, and Kevin Orr
on staff, was doing a good job on AIDS education and prevention work
with affected communities.[22]

"Ruthless interference with our bereavement"

Shortly after the Jarvis meeting, Lynch made another trip to New
York, staying with Spiers. Lynch went to see *Les Misérables* with his
friend Michael Jorgensen: *"He cries over empty tables, empty chairs
(the survivors song) I over the Valjean father to 'son' song—'Bring him
home.'"* Lynch also presented a paper at New York University and
met with a representative of Contact II Publications, which wanted
to publish a volume of his poetry.

Sitting in a coffee shop on Park Avenue, Lynch wrote in his diary
about a front-page article in *The New York Times*. The newspaper was
already infamous in the gay community for its lack of AIDS coverage
during the early years of the epidemic. Lynch had just read a Sunday
edition feature that reported on the epidemic as being over because
the illness wasn't spreading into the "general population," and not
spreading much among gays. It was spreading among IV drug users,
but then, *"they don't count, or travel,"* Lynch wrote. In its wisdom the
paper conceded that many deaths were still to come among the
already infected: one-half of the gay men in San Francisco would die,
and one-quarter of gay men in the United States as a whole. *"But the
message, the main message, was this: 'we are saved.'"*

Douglas Crimp, art critic and ACT UP member, captured the emotional impact of that kind of article, which assumes a reader not
directly affected by the epidemic: "For anyone living daily with the
AIDS crisis, ruthless interference with our bereavement is as ordinary
an occurrence as reading the *New York Times*."[23]

Lynch had decided to stop taking AZT at the beginning of February,
when fatigue made it difficult for him to complete a lecture. He had

already had five blood transfusions to combat the anaemia that was a common side effect of the drug. By the time he went to New York he had been off AZT for almost two weeks, and was low in every sense— *"including spirits, energy, haematology, hope and fortitude."* For the first time ever, he noted, the conversations he and Herb were having *assumed* that neither one of them would be a survivor.

Lynch also went to see New York doctor Howard Grossman. After hearing of Lynch's difficulties with AZT, Grossman prescribed Antabuse, which was usually prescribed for heavy drinkers of alcohol who wanted to quit. It became an underground treatment for PWAS in the late 1980s because it had a similar structure to a drug, Imuthiol, which was reported to be an immune modulator but was not available in North America. Shortly after that, in Toronto, some of Lynch's students asked him out for a beer after class. Lynch declined, saying he was on Antabuse. *"No doubt they think I'm an alcoholic. O.K. So be it."*

Spiers was just then completing a presentation, on behalf of ACT UP, to President Ronald Reagan's Commission on AIDS. When he delivered it, on February 19, 1988, Lynch was in the audience. Spiers emphasized the dismal state of AIDS drug testing in the United States. In the entire country there was only one drug trial under the AIDS Treatment and Evaluation Unit (ATEU) Program that was testing a drug other than AZT, and there were only twenty-five slots open to patients in that trial. The ATEU had been set up by the National Institute of Allergy and Infectious Diseases to facilitate clinical trials into AIDS drugs. Spiers told the committee that his mistake, like that of other people affected by AIDS, was:

> to remain silent too long; quiet in the assumption that the health of the body politic was above the ideological issues of partisan politics. With our mouths closed, we watched the deaths mount. . . . Sad to say, in the Age of AIDS, many of us have learned that in our democratic society, the price of health is perpetual pressure and an ever ready pair of vocal cords.[24]

Lynch also went to see John Huston's movie *The Dead* in New York, and he wept profusely, early on in the film, when he saw Huston's camera caressing the face and head, *"the whole dressed body,"* of the director's daughter, Angelica Huston. *"This movie is a love poem from father to grown daughter. Stress 'grown.' How I'd love to be around to see Stefan grown to that age."* Lynch, too, had been concerned that Stefan had not yet mourned for Bill Lewis, who had been a stepfather to him, so he was relieved to hear that both Stefan and Gail had begun separate support groups. Stefan had his worst fears confirmed—that his father was HIV-positive—only by overhearing his father tell someone on the telephone.

Back in Toronto after his brief New York visit, Lynch found himself dealing with a distraught son. Stefan wanted to come home to his father. In his combined grief over Bill and fears for his father, Stefan decided he should quit San Rafael immediately and move to 8 Ross. Gail and Lynch talked and decided to say "no"—please finish out the year at San Rafael. Lynch was left wondering about how to find ways of working on Stefan's fear that one day his father would "suddenly" be dying. *"Rationality doesn't help. I can explain the different situation of BL and me, the stats, the reasons for greater longevity—but the lesson of Bill's death won't be untaught. Poor Stefan—in fact, I'd love to have him here at 8 Ross, we'd enjoy each other a lot."* But in the end he felt that Stefan changing school *"in the middle of a storm"* would be a bad idea.

Randy Coates, the epidemiologist who had been a good friend of Bill Lewis, called to say he had tested HIV-positive. Coates told very few people and, given his academic discipline and his own research into AIDS, was mortified about the test results, said his friend Sarah Yates-Howorth. According to Lynch, Coates was also anxious because there had recently been a controversy over the idea of placing practice restrictions on health-care workers infected with HIV.[25]

After Lynch chaired an AAN! meeting that worked on a constitution for the organization and planned a demonstration for late March, he commented, *"George Smith is so **soothing** as a political confrere; he eases my tortuosities."* Lynch's last entry for diary number 57 came on March 10, 1988. His last line: *"Will I live through #58?"*

Coffins in the rain: a placebo strike

On March 25, AAN! staged its first demonstration, organized by Kinsman and McCaskell when Lynch was out of town. The target of the protest was the lack of availability of aerosolized pentamidine in Canada. McCaskell had a friend, Akio Nakajima, who was dying in hospital and was denied aerosolized pentamidine. Nakajimi was being treated with the much more toxic intravenous form of the drug, which was causing seizures. "It took me an hour to convince a doctor that something was really wrong," said McCaskell. He asked the doctors why Nakajimi couldn't receive the pentamidine in an aerosolized form, and they just said, "Sorry, we can't do that." McCaskell, angry, knew that he had to take some kind of action.[26]

AAN! was also protesting that the clinical trials of the drug being contemplated for Canada involved placebos. In a randomized controlled trial (RCT), the gold standard for research, some participants would be given the drug and some would be given a placebo—a so-called "sugar" pill with no active ingredients—as a means of ascertaining the effects of the drug. The activists argued that because it was known that a certain number of those taking placebos would go on to develop PCP, a life-threatening illness, and because the drug had already been shown to be effective in preventing PCP when used by some doctors in the United States, the use of a placebo was unethical. In late 1987 in New York, the newly formed Community Research Initiative had begun its own trials of aerosolized pentamidine, as had a similar group in San Francisco.[27] These trials compared different doses of aerosolized pentamidine, without using placebos. Randomized controlled trials made perfect sense from a researcher's point of view, but not from the point of view of the research subject with AIDS.

"It's one thing to have people die from this epidemic. It's another to have people die because of some stupid government regulation that says people can't get drugs that people elsewhere are using," McCaskell said.[28]

Patients like Alan Dewar, who had already suffered through two bouts of PCP, were not eligible for the trial, because only those who had experienced only one bout of PCP qualified. "People at most severe risk of redeveloping PCP will have to wait months until the study is finished," Dewar said. Just over a week later, Fisons, the drug company conducting the trial, introduced a "compassionate arm," under which people who had already had two bouts of pneumonia could get pentamidine just by signing up.[29]

Among those who had joined AAN! were several Toronto visual artists, and their influence on the organization's protests quickly became apparent. About five hundred marchers began in the rain at the 519 Community Centre on Church Street. At the front of the procession, demonstrators carried three empty coffins, representing the three or four people who would, predictably, die unless the placebo part of a planned trial of aerosolized pentamidine was cancelled. "Remember that what we're doing is marching to *keep* them empty," McCaskell told CBC-Radio.[30] AAN! called the protest action a "placebo strike."

The protest wound through downtown Toronto, making a stop outside the office of David Crombie, Conservative MP for the area (Rosedale). Earlier on, an AAN! member had been dispatched to buy red duct tape to stick on Crombie's office door, and now Lynch gave a passionate speech decrying the red tape that held back drug therapies for PWAS. The protest culminated with a candlelight vigil outside the Toronto General Hospital, one of the sites slated for the aerosolized pentamidine drug trial.

The protest was widely covered by the local media, and represented a significant change in the depiction of AIDS for readers and viewers. Until that time, mainstream media coverage in Toronto had focused on mortality statistics and dying victims. But these marchers were angry. AAN! had an official policy of declining government or corporate money (except on occasion for a specific project), and it raised $900 at the demo. Its July financial statement itemized expenses: $58.50 for candles and $72.38 for lumber for the coffins.

Dissension and democracy

Not everyone in Toronto's gay community was thrilled with AAN!'s approach. Randy Coates, who helped found ACT, was *"utterly enraged by AAN!'s methods and persuaded the ACT board not to support the demo,"* Lynch wrote. And ACT chair Art Wood, during a lunch meeting with Lynch before the March 25 demo, trashed an AAN! brochure produced to promote the event and criticized the decision to target the Toronto General Hospital rather than the Federal Centre for AIDS. Wood told Lynch, who had recently become the first chair of AAN!, that he was *"a chair being chaired"* by others in the organization. Wood's criticisms did not have the desired effect: *"Since I am eager **not** to chair in an executive fashion, more in a facilitating fashion, I was quite pleased with the latter comment,"* Lynch told his diary. He had been impressed by the style of ACT UP meetings that he had attended in New York. "They were so exciting," recalled Jackson, who attended some of the same meetings. "They were run very democratically— you'd have two to three strong people, a couple of men and a woman would chair these things. But they were free for alls, because they didn't have a tight organization. They didn't have funding except what was donated to them, so there really was a sense that they didn't have to set up all these structures . . . it was democracy on the floor of the lesbian and gay community and it was a very exciting sort of thing."

Over the days before and after the March 25 demonstration, Lynch was criticized for several "acts of politics," and he wrote that, indeed, in some areas, he could have made more considered decisions. *"But I might also have lost energy, infusion, initiative. And just now, that would have been too great a price to pay. Initiative!"*

The candlelight vigil outside Toronto General Hospital during the March 25 demonstration *"had an unplanned private click!"* for Lynch. Six months earlier the hospital had been the site of the silent support circle that he had convened outside Lewis's hospital room. *"Well, it wasn't quite silent at TGH,"* he wrote in a diary entry addressed to Lewis. *"People sang 'We Shall Overcome' (I'm sure you groaned) and the lugubrious 'We are a gay and gentle people.' Russell* [Armstrong] *proposed afterwards that we commission a new gay anthem by someone."*

When he spoke with a bullhorn outside Crombie's constituency office, Lynch said he *"felt a gap between my ideology and level of anger, level of emotion and the crowd's. There was a coolness and detachment in the tone that made it different from American demos I've been to."* He attributed it to Canadian "emotional lassitude." But others who were there remember only that Lynch delivered a powerful and inspiring speech. In his diary Lynch queried some of the facts that McCaskell gave in his speech and Tim's characterization of placebo trials as "evil." But, Lynch concluded, *"In the streets, the facts can be looser—as long as in the policy papers and on the TV debates they're tight. Nevertheless I'm a stickler, as I am a fusser over political mishaps. Tim may be amused at my worry . . . lest we walk right past ACT* [at 464 Yonge Street] *if the crowd was in an anti-ACT mood. But they weren't, we did, and he may."* Given what he'd seen going on in New York, Lynch was no doubt particularly sensitive to the risk of hostilities between the service organization and the activist one.

When he read *The Toronto Star* and *The Globe and Mail* the next day, Lynch felt "very small." The papers only just barely covered the demo. Gary Kinsman, though, said he found the demonstration significant because the fledgling organization had managed to pull together "a credible demo that people found quite moving, that symbolized what was going on, and that put pressure on those conducting [aerosolized pentamidine] trials and on drug release in general."

And there were some rewards for Lynch. He spotted one of his American fiction students in the crowd at the TGH vigil: *"There is a pleasure these days that I'm a **gay** leader/thinker to some of my gay students, male and female,"* he told his diary. *"Of course I want to be loved, admired, pedestalled, beatified. I also want to keep kicking against the pricks and all canonization."*

In a letter to AAN!'s public action committee, Lynch urged members to keep up the momentum. He suggested a series of projects, including actions against Fisons and other pharmaceutical companies, Jake Epp, Alastair Clayton, and Bay Street, and a walk to Buffalo, as a way of symbolizing the aerosolized pentamidine issue.[31]

AAN!'s strength, like that of ACT UP, was its ability to channel anger and enthusiasm into a push for access to treatment for PWAS. These goals were urgent—many members were already infected and ailing. Right from the beginning, AAN! had to cope with continuing deaths among its members. Within the first two years of its existence, the organization would lose key members, among them Alan Dewar (who died October 4, 1988, at forty-four years of age), James McPhee (November 39, 1989, twenty-six), Chuck Grochmal (February 3, 1990, thirty-seven), and Graham Campbell (January 17, 1990, thirty-six).

When he was at the March on Washington in October 1987, Lynch had seen both the Vietnam Memorial and the AIDS Quilt. Those two grassroots memorials—the Vietnam Memorial was paid for with money raised by veterans, and the AIDS Quilt was made by lovers, family, and friends of PWAS—no doubt influenced his desire to see a similar installation in Canada and planted the seeds for his next big project, an AIDS memorial. During a Christmas 1987 visit to California, Lynch also had long discussions with gay historian Allan Bérubé, who had made his own video of the AIDS Quilt and encouraged Lynch's efforts to "enact common mourning." In an article he wrote on the subject, Bérubé spoke of the importance of grieving in the face of randomness; and, subsequently, the importance of turning grief into action.[32]

Lynch's article "The Power of Names: Finding Ways to Remember Our Friends" was published in *Xtra* in February 1988:

> With the wave of local funerals over the last six months, I have a hunch that downtown Toronto gays have recently reached a critical mass: AIDS is our problem, for real now. The deaths of widely known people such as Andy Armstrong, Don Barlow and Jim Saar bring home the news, even if we don't yet have private friends on our lists. Are we ready for a communal naming, for once and all, to replace those dehumanizing numbers? . . . An old cliché motivates me a lot these days. It goes: "That they shall not have died in vain."[33]

On April 14 Lynch met with Jacques D'Angenais, a teacher at the Ontario College of Art, and asked him to design an AIDS memorial for Toronto. As it happened, the Toronto AIDS Memorial would begin life as a temporary structure—like the quilt, it was brought out for certain occasions—and ended up as a permanent wall of names, not unlike the Vietnam Memorial.

Lynch's life was once again a whirlwind of activity, from one meeting to another, from AAN! work to the *Gay Studies Newsletter*, from the AIDS memorial to a benefit for the Canadian Gay archives featuring film historian Vito Russo. *"O.k., I'm this way, driven,"* Lynch told his diary.

Two days after meeting with D'Angenais Lynch gave a paper, based on his "Age of Adhesiveness" work, at the first Lesbian and Gay Studies Conference at the City University of New York. In the midst of all this scholarly activity, the June 1988 issue of the U.S. gay skin magazine *Mandate* was published (in early May), featuring several pages of erotic photographs of Lynch. "He had to be the only university professor, gay activist, poet porn star," laughed his friend Robert Wallace. *"Gives me a little sense of physicality again—and that particular energy of seeking myself as a public 'himself,'"* Lynch wrote in his diary. *"For a queen in her 40s, he doesn't look half bad either . . . How Lynch is fortunate. He seems to get so many of the things he wants, and leads a rich life: silly, impactful, sober, indulgent—all at once.* Mandate *and* These Waves*! Billy, are you giggling too?"*[34]

Broken promises and the Royal Society

In April AAN! began publishing its own newsletter, which would come out every two, three, or four months for the next six years. The initial issue included an article tracing the history of the federal government's broken promises to PWAS, including a mention of the trip made to Ottawa in June 1986 by Kevin Brown and Warren Jensen to urge release of experiment drugs to PWAS. In October that same year Health Minister Epp had pledged that the Health Protection Branch would seek out, encourage the availability, and facilitate the use of experimental drugs in Canada, adding that "everything possible will be done by the Health Protection Branch to facilitate the whole process."[35] It was a hollow promise. In late 1986 a limited number of PWAS in Canada became eligible for AZT (at the time, estimates were that 150 to 180 people would qualify). In March 1987, the Food and Drug Administration in the United States approved AZT for use by the 33,000 Americans who had been diagnosed with AIDS, while in Canada, two months later, the federal government allowed the sale of AZT only to selected qualified investigators for clinical testing in what was referred to as an "open clinical trial."[36] But in 1988 no other experimental drugs were available for PWAS in the country.

On March 13, 1988, Lynch took his first dose of a three-month supply of Dextran Sulphate, another promising drug that AAN! wanted to see undergoing clinical trials in Canada along with Ampligen and Antabuse. Dextran Sulphate had been available without a prescription in Japan for years, and that's where Lynch understood his supply had come from. It was originally intended for a New York friend, Ken Calendar, but Calendar was *"too out of things with* [AIDS] *dementia to take it."* In fact, the only North American manufacturer of the substance was located right in Metropolitan Toronto, in Scarborough. But federal officials blocked distribution of the substance on the basis that because it was touted as something to fight AIDS, it would have to be approved as a drug and could not be sold without prescription as a nutritional supplement. "I understand the attempts to shield Canadians from chemicals that can cause them harm," said Dr. Denis Conway of AAN!—"but those who have catastrophic illnesses feel they have nothing to lose and everything to gain by taking an experimental drug."[37]

AAN! wasn't the only body casting a critical eye over the federal government's record on AIDS. In spring 1988 the Royal Society of Canada completed its report *AIDS: A Perspective for Canadians*, commissioned by the Medical Research Council and the federal Department of Health and Welfare.[38] The Society, whose members included scientists and academics, called for Ottawa to increase its research funding by seven times, from the $4.26 million allocated in 1987–88 to at least $35 million a year. "Greatly increased levels of clinical research are essential," stated the report, which also urged Ottawa to establish a liaison with the U.S. National Institutes of Health to allow Canadian participation in new drug trials. The authors of the report were adamant that ad hoc care for people living with AIDS was no longer defensible. The report also called for $80 million a year to be spent on education around AIDS. It provoked controversy by suggesting that governments in Canada distribute free condoms and provide needle-sterilizing facilities for people, including prisoners and injection drug users, engaged in activities that risk the spread of AIDS. "If reason points that way, then why defy reason and refuse to do the sensible thing in preventing the spread of the risk?" asked Mr. Justice Horace Krever, one of the thirty-four volunteer contributors to the report.[39]

Getting attention: sex, danger, conflict—and illegal drugs

The Sheraton Hotel is in the heart of downtown Toronto, directly across Queen Street West from City Hall and its plaza, Nathan Phillips Square. Still dubbed "new," the striking oyster-shell-like towers of City Hall were built in 1965 and designed by Finnish architect Viljo Revell. They sit across Bay Street from "old" City Hall, now a courthouse. It was at the Sheraton that the third Canadian Conference on AIDS was to be held on May 16 and 17, 1988. The meeting was co-sponsored by the Canadian Public Health Association, the Federal Centre for AIDS, and the Canadian AIDS Society, which held its own annual meeting on May 14–15.

CAS had been formally established in November 1986, with sixteen founding members. The national organization was created largely in order to provide the federal government with a central body that it could connect to in its approaches to AIDS. As well, AIDS service organizations (ASOs) that were having trouble obtaining provincial funding, like AIDS Vancouver, became eligible for federal money through the national organization. By the time of the Sheraton meeting, CAS comprised thirty-one large and small ASOs from across Canada, and there was much discontent in the ranks. Members of the National Advisory Committee on AIDS were also disgruntled. One member told the conference that the Committee could not afford to meet. At the time the Committee, starved of funds, had not met for six months.[40]

AAN! planned to disrupt the proceedings with a combined inside and outside operation. Kinsman, Greg Pavelich, and another AAN! member got inside the conference on Monday, May 16, and during a speech by Maureen Law, the federal deputy minister of health, they unfurled and silently held up a banner reading "EPP = DEATH." Epp had been particularly unresponsive both to PWAS around treatment issues and to the needs of ASOs. Epp did not attend the conference. The only elected officials present were Toronto city councillor Jack Layton and a councillor from Ottawa.

Outside the hotel, AAN! members organized a "die-in" to symbolize where the politics of the federal government were leading with respect to AIDS and HIV. "A government which denies Canadians drug access is a government which contributes to the deaths of Canadians," Lynch told the gathering. "It's a shameless government that fires one minister because of some tainted tuna but retains one whose policy actively threatens the lives of 30,000" (the estimated number of HIV-infected Canadians).[41]

At the close of the conference the next day, AAN! organizers were gratified to see conference participants swell the ranks of a late afternoon demonstration. About three hundred protestors gathered outside the hotel and then marched along Richmond Street, briefly taking it over and blocking traffic, before moving along to the regional offices of the federal Progressive Conservative Party. There they "stuck their demands on the door: Epp's resignation and action from the Federal Centre for AIDS."[42] They then marched back to Nathan Phillips Square. Kinsman, one of the marshals for the protest, was delighted that people from ASOs across the country had joined in. There was a growing recognition, he thought, that government policies, pharmaceutical policies, and certain members of the medical profession were preventing people from gaining access to drugs that would extend their lives. "People were experiencing a very direct contradiction: there were these treatments, and there were social forces standing in their way," Kinsman said. Police were ready to stop the protestors from gathering at the square, because they didn't have a permit. "Fortunately, Metro councillor Jack Layton was marching with us and told the police we were his guests," George Smith wrote later. "They let us in—but not before councillor Layton had to produce his ID."[43]

Lynch made the central speech to the crowd. "Canadians do not want a health minister who lets their sons, daughters, and lovers die. AIDS is no longer a sentence to immediate death. We want drugs that will help us live." Michael Davis of the Federal Centre for AIDS told *The Globe and Mail*, "I understand the frustration, but I really wonder what they want. There's really nothing much out there that might do any good, only unproven drugs that can be taken out of desperation."[44]

Leading the crowd in chanting, Lynch yelled out something about how far away Ottawa was geographically and politically and that they weren't going to hear them in Ottawa at that level of noise. "So he got people making a whole lot of noise, which was echoing wonderfully at City Hall," Glen Brown said. Brown also clearly recalled Lynch saying that "as an educator, he was loathe to write off anybody as someone who could not learn, but he concluded that Jake Epp was *ineducable*"—a word Brown had never heard before. Lynch's remark was probably a reference to Epp's own statements about AIDS education programs having very little effect. Canadians have a high level of awareness about AIDS, Epp said in January 1988. "But the level of knowledge does not change the behaviour of high-risk groups, and we so far have limited evidence of how much change in high-risk groups has taken place." At the time, there had in fact been a significant drop in the rate of sexually transmitted diseases among gay men in the United States and Canada.[45]

Stephen Manning, executive director of ACT, spoke to the crowd and endorsed the protest action—an unusual step for an organization concerned about jeopardizing its government funding and charitable status. "When people are facing catastrophic illnesses, we need new rules," he told the crowd. The government "says it can't release new drugs because they might hurt us, but what we have is killing us."[46]

But it was the burning of a full-size effigy of Epp that captured the media's—and the government's—attention and propelled AAN! onto the national stage. "Burn the dummy!" and "Fire Epp!" were the rallying cries as the protestors gathered at City Hall. *"Police were not amused, but did little to interfere. The media were delighted and recorded everything,"* Lynch told his diary. He summarized what had happened in four days of work: AIDS issues had become a national issue, and AAN! actions had made all three national TV network evenings news for two nights running. *"Bill, I hear you giggle at what we're accomplishing."* That evening Lynch, Alan Miller, Gram Campbell, and Kevin Brown had come back to the house and "devoured" three pizzas. *"I looked up at the urn and at your picture and missed you and felt how you motivate me."*

"We couldn't have asked for a better media landscape," Glen Brown said of those times. "We were the first people to talk about AIDS as a political issue, and AIDS itself was a hot issue. It had all the elements of a great news story—sex and danger and conflict—but having said that, we certainly exploited that landscape very well, very effectively. And folks like Michael were adept at that."

George Smith, writing in the gay and lesbian tabloid *Rites*, noted that the media reported the AAN!-organized demonstration as the work of the entire AIDS conference being held at the Sheraton Hotel. "It was really great that AAN!'s activist politics struck such a resounding chord and were able to focus, in a public way, the real concerns of PLWAS and AIDS workers . . . it was also clear that people across the country felt very deeply about the government's lack of leadership on AIDS treatments."[47]

For some of the people who worked at AIDS service organizations and joined in the protest, burning an effigy of the health minister was a "pretty radical act," recalled Jackson. And the events in Toronto had an immediate impact in Ottawa. A couple of weeks later Epp was called into Prime Minister Brian Mulroney's office and asked about just what it was that the minister was doing or not doing that was making people in Toronto so angry. Some of the answers to that question had become apparent at the CAS annual meeting. Member organizations complained about a lack of support and communication from the federal government, and reported about homophobic and disturbing attitudes and actions by some provincial governments. For example, the Nova Scotia health minister had suggested quarantine for sexually active people with AIDS, and British Columbia had introduced a bill that would have given the government power to quarantine anyone suspected of testing positive for antibodies to HIV.[48]

Indeed, in both Nova Scotia and British Columbia elected officials had considered designating islands off the coasts—former leper colonies—as quarantine sites for people with AIDS, noted Douglas Elliott, a lawyer who represented the Canadian AIDS Society during the Commission of Inquiry on the Blood System in Canada. CAS was involved in the Krever inquiry in part to help document the early AIDS movement and initiatives in the gay community. Elliott was told of a push inside the B.C. government to "put a wall around the west end [in Vancouver] and round up all AIDS carriers." In Saskatchewan CAS uncovered a request for funding sent by an AIDS group to the Saskatchewan health minister. The document had been found in the minister's files with "Go to Hell" scribbled over it. Elliott said that across the country the pattern varied: "Sometimes we saw that public health officials were entreating homophobic [provincial government] ministers to do something; sometimes we saw elected officials being thwarted or stymied by homophobic bureaucrats."

In March 1988, British Columbia decided not to cover the costs of AZT, and people who had been taking the drug received huge bills retroactive to the summer of 1987.[49] (The annual cost for the drug was about $11,000 per person, and every other province paid for AZT for people with HIV/AIDS.) Meanwhile, Marvin Moore, Alberta's minister of hospitals, argued that provincial medical research money should go to Alzheimer's disease and cancer, but not to AIDS, because AIDS was more "preventable." Ontario was somewhat more progressive. In spring 1988 it launched a two-year $7 million advertising and information campaign about AIDS. The target, though, was the general population. Gay men were not mentioned at all, and IV drug users only once.[50]

Fresh from the success of the Toronto demonstration, AAN! kept up the pressure. A little more than a week later, on May 25, another media event dreamed up by Lynch drew attention to the issues, making headlines and newscasts across the country. Lynch and fellow PWAS Bill Greenway, Chuck Grochmal, and James Thomas sat in front of the Peace Tower at the Parliament Buildings in Ottawa and took AIDS drugs that had not yet been approved for use in Canada. Greenway inhaled aerosolized pentamidine, Lynch took Naltrexone, Thomas took Dextran Sulphate, and Grochmal took AL-721, a promising antiviral drug developed in Israel. Protestors behind them carried signs declaring "Placebos Equal Death." The entire event was staged to play off the clock at the top of the Peace Tower and illustrate the urgency of treatment needs for people with AIDS.

Before the event at the Peace Tower, protestors had demonstrated at the Federal Centre for AIDS, located at the corner of Elgin and McLaren, and then marched along Elgin Street to the National Press Theatre to hold a press conference. Dr. Alastair Clayton, head of the Federal Centre, joined the march. "The man who has done more than most to obstruct treatment for PLWAS tried to pretend that he was for AIDS Action Now! What hypocrisy!" George Smith wrote in

Rites.[51] Lynch, along with Smith and other AAN! leaders, decided to decline a last-minute invitation from the government for what he termed a token audience. The decision *"makes me feel like a wild card, and that's as it should be."* Instead, he flew back from Ottawa in time to teach a 6 p.m. class on *Uncle Tom's Cabin*.

Waking up in the middle of the night a few days later, Lynch scribbled out lyrics for an AIDS anthem in *"a world war 2 marching song style."* The song began:

> *Act up [act up] fight back [fight back]*
> *We want AIDS action now*
> *No more stalling, no more lies*
> *no more pity, we want life . . .*

"Shit, I didn't have any staff paper to write down the tune before going back to sleep," Lynch wrote the next morning. *"Tried to fix it in my ears—but (except for a little) I lost it."* Apparently, Lynch dropped the idea. AAN! never did get its own anthem.

Meanwhile, plans for the AIDS Memorial were proceeding. Jacques D'Angenais's show and tell, outlining colours, fabrics, and lettering style, made Lynch teary. The tears came, he wrote, because *"my original idea 1) would get realized and 2) would get realized at a far higher pitch of quality than I'd imagined, even."*

On June 8 Epp announced that Ottawa would grant $129 million towards AIDS over the next five years. The money, to be administered and distributed by the Federal Centre for AIDS, was allocated to education, research, prevention and care, training for health-care workers, program and policy development, and international AIDS actions. The next day, on a morning television program with Epp, Lynch pointed out that the minister's funding announcement added up to only $26 million a year, compared to the $115 million a year that the Royal Society had recommended in April for research and education. The Federal Centre, he argued, should be "investigated, not funded." He noted that the Royal Society, in its report on what Canada should do about AIDS, did not even mention the Centre, an omission that underscored the institution's lack of importance.[52]

Canada's drug approval system was simply not up to the challenge of AIDS—particularly the challenge of making new drugs available. Clayton told reporters that the Federal Centre was "looking at" several new AIDS drugs, including Dextran Sulphate and ddC (dideoxy-cytidine). The drug ddC, like AZT and ddI (dideoxyinosine), belonged to the family of drugs known as nucleoside analogues. It was showing promise in U.S. clinical trials, but no Canadian trials of it and the other drugs were being contemplated, and Canadian participation in U.S. trials—as recommended in the Royal Society report—had not been considered. Indeed, when Michael Hulton went, on his own, to the U.S. National Institutes of Health in the spring of 1988, he was told that Canadian officials were simply not coming to visit the U.S. AIDS research headquarters. He was also told that the NIH was prepared, at least in theory, to have Canadians participate in their drug trials.

Bureaucrats just didn't seem to understand—or were ignoring—the urgency of the situation and the need to change some of the rules. Dr. Norbert Gilmore diagnosed the problem:

> The difficulty we're dealing with is it's a system that was set up to be careful about drugs—for instance drugs for hypertension, other infections and so on, like that—where they could really be evaluated before they just went out there and started being used. Now suddenly we're on to a sort of pressure cooker where they need to be done immediately.

Gilmore pointed out that a great many people now needed the drugs immediately, and everyone involved had to figure out some way of delivering them. "And I don't think we've been able to do that yet, and that's the problem."[53]

Stephen Manning of ACT put it more succinctly: "We think that when people are facing catastrophic illness, you have to have different rules. This is not like trying to get a licence for a new brand of aspirin."[54]

eight

THE CHARM OF POLITICS

DURING THE SUMMER of 1988 Michael Lynch was still the chair of AIDS Action Now! and a guiding force in the organization. He sent memos, handled a lot of media contacts, and consulted with fellow activists. But he wasn't attending very many meetings. In mid-September Tim McCaskell took over as chair of the organization.

It was a familiar pattern. Lynch had been the catalyst behind many important initiatives in the gay and lesbian community in Toronto; but most of the time, as soon as he felt that a new organization or project was well launched, he withdrew from day-to-day involvement. His energies were just as quickly absorbed with the next project. That summer he had two other endeavours—the AIDS Memorial and the Toronto Centre for Lesbian and Gay Studies.

"The charm of politics is that someone is always there to tell you you're wrong," he told his diary in late June 1988.

I'm fond of those who criticize your strategy by assuming you had no strategy, of those with leisure to read books and look up from time to time to make the historical arguments. Resentment comes easily when you've worked your ass off and people still sitting on theirs call you one, even though, having worked it off, you don't have one any more. The irony is simple: I hate all politicians, myself included, and love politics (and hate it that I do): my ear a cauliflower, my French more broken than ever, my friends wondering if they'll ever see me again, but, sometimes, something gets done. I miss not spending an

> hour with, say, a good A major scale, until the thumb passes under
> and wrist pirouettes so that to the ear both thumb and wrist are
> absent, only A major **is**. I miss reading, and that I'll die without hav-
> ing read Cervantes, or Mary Shelly or Marquez, if only to see what
> the fuss is about. Or rereading the all male court scene in the middle
> of As You Like It, or rereading Proust. I miss reading my contempo-
> raries, whether I like them or not, in order to have time for phone
> calls and sealing envelopes and pulling together lawyers, like Lego,
> for committee. I miss leisurely hot summer evenings when you drop
> in unannounced at the neighbours who are rocking in rocking chairs
> on their porches and who actually **welcome** you with iced tea.
> Sometimes you give up a lot for politics, most often without making
> a choice in full conscience. Sometimes, you half regret what you've
> given up in order to chair meetings. But sometimes, something gets
> done.

Things do get done: less than a week later, at one in the morning on
Lesbian and Gay Pride Day 1988, Lynch was writing in his diary: *"In
5 hours, the memorial begins to go up. It's windy now; I'm jittery. What a
few months ago was a wisp in my little imagination is soon to be 'real.'
Never experienced anything like that before."* After a few hours of sleep,
Lynch joined several others at Cawthra Park, adjacent to the 519
Community Centre on Church Street, in the area that had, since the
early 1980s, developed into the city's gay ghetto. It was Sunday, June
26. *"We gathered at the park at 6, rolled out the rubbies (the class function of the park found its timetable moved by 3 hours) . . . And the native
homeless yielded to the white middle classes, who picked up the empty
hootch bottles to substitute, later, their own cigarette butts. Twenty people did the building and we finished early."*

Lynch's friend Gerald Hannon, in a magazine article published
later that year, wrote of that first memorial: "We all joke that it is as
tasteful as only a dedicated group of homosexual decorators could
make it. Inside, past the great vases of flowers at the entrance, you
wander down a quiet hallway of pale greens and blues and mauves,
of soft earth colours set off by the startling white of support ropes, by
evergreens, by the achingly blue sky. Each panel carries a list of names,
each name carefully inscribed in silver ink on a small placard."[1]

The memorial was officially opened at noon. With television cameras rolling, Lynch began reading the names of the dead. Another

reader was Martin, a young man in his mid-twenties whose father had died a few months earlier. Martin, an only child, was eager to participate in the reading, Lynch wrote. *"A son surviving a father, with much much tenderness and completeness"*—his participation had a great appeal for Lynch. There were two hundred names on the memorial when it was unveiled. By 7 p.m., when it was closed to be dismantled, another hundred names had been added. The numbers were small given that at least twelve hundred people had died of AIDS in Canada—the toll would be 1,790 by the end of 1988—but relatives or friends had to submit names to be included in the memorial.

"People bunched and crowded in the memorial early in the afternoon," Lynch wrote, but after the Pride Day parade *"they filed through slowly, almost single file, with such barely held in emotions (it **is** Ontario) I cried a lot just watching others cry."* Lynch ripped part of a page out of the Pride Day booklet, a headline that said "Community," and stuck it by Bill Lewis's name on the memorial, later tucking a condom there as well. *"How I want you back. How I wanted you there yesterday, kvetching and happy and sparkly and with a bit of a belly under your sleeveless T,"* Lynch wrote, in a diary entry addressed, once again, to Bill.

The idea behind the memorial was to create a place for private and communal mourning, but Lynch acknowledged that he would have liked some credit for his initiative—that his "ego needed stroking" for his work on the memorial. *"I've an American ego wanting American strokes."* He observed that U.S. activist Cleve Jones had received acclaim for his work promoting the AIDS Quilt south of the border. *"But in Canada we don't lionize. And of course Americans pay no attention to **anything** Canadians do."*

Bad dreams: mourning and activism

A few days later, on a visit to Eve Kosofsky Sedgwick in Amherst, Massachusetts, Lynch was disturbed by a dream.

> *In this hateful dream, I am in charge of an aids demonstration. We will be carrying real caskets with real bodies in them. Over the last week, we have stored perhaps 20 bodies to use for this demo. They are stored in large file drawers in offices on an upper floor of a tall*

office building. We have come to remove them for the demo. But we forgot: it is 5:00, it is Friday, and tonight is Halloween. No one is leaving the offices, because all are having Halloween office parties. Furthermore, the elevators are clogged with people going down floor to floor in costume. The occasion frustrates us—people still around— but might also help us—if the coffins could appear to be party props. We try, but the removal of each body takes far more time than we'd allowed for. I get jumpy; when do we begin the demo? We have gotten about 12 of the 20 bodies, & though I don't know what will happen to the other 8, I decide we must begin now. Dream over.[2]

The dream echoed through the following day when, at an electronic shop, he spotted a VCR with a repair tag on it. Under the category "trouble," someone had specified "dead." Later, during a tour of Emily Dickinson's home, an insensitive tour guide didn't cite any of the poet's writing and, Lynch wrote, *"Everything is keeping her away from me."* That evening, showing Kosofsky Sedgwick a videotape of the CBC-TV special on "AIDS and the Arts" that he had participated in, he observed, *"I now see it is about death and dying, not about AIDS."*

Stefan was back in Toronto for the summer and at the end of June joined his father for what they called "the dead authors tour" of New England. The two of them flew to Boston and rented a car and spent a week driving around to the graves of Lynch's favourite nine-teenth-century authors—Dickinson, Herman Melville, and Louisa May Alcott—in places like Concord and Lexington. For a teenager, as Stefan put it, the whole idea of the trip "was brutal." One of the places Michael wanted to go was Arrowhead, to see Melville's house, the place where the great author had written *Moby Dick.* "To my Dad's absolute shock it was about 150 miles inland." His father, Stefan added, "had a vision of a house on the ocean where Melville transcribed what he saw, and I remember laughing at how shocked he was."

Stefan was hating his Marin County, California, high school. After writing the Student Achievement Tests (SATs) and obtaining a high score, he was inundated with mail from colleges urging him to consider them after high school. One piece of mail, from Simon's Rock College of Bard, in Great Barrington, Massachusetts, asked,

"Why wait to go to college?" That, thought Stefan, was a damn good question. During the dead authors tour Stefan and Lynch visited Simon's Rock, a college that accepted students who had completed Grade 10, and both of them fell in love with it. Stefan applied and was accepted later in the summer. It was a fateful decision, as Stefan explained a decade after his father's death.

> I had two and a half years of college before my Dad died, and he related differently to me once I was in college. That was his life, university, the language and all sorts of things he was comfortable with. So it really changed our connection. . . . He could relate to me on the plane he was comfortable with, he could talk to me about ideas and literature and about the kinds of things that he was used to talking to peers about.

Back in Toronto, Lynch received a package of the monotype illustrations that Douglas Kinsey had created to accompany the poems in a book that Contact II Publications of New York had agreed to publish. The artwork was black, literally and figuratively. *"Of course I am 'dark' & have much of my years been devoted to moving there, to being it, to living with loss and as a mourner,"* Lynch wrote. *"I know all this, but take it for granted. And am surprised when a reader/listener/painter-or-critic registers the obvious."*

With flagging energy, which he pegged at about 30 per cent of his normal level, Lynch nonetheless enrolled in a conversational French class that summer. He had done several interviews for AAN! with the Quebec media, and had been inspired to improve his fluency. He already had some French; he had spent part of a year living and studying in France while he was an undergraduate.

After attending yet another AIDS funeral (for Mark deWolfe, a friend of Lewis's who had been a Unitarian minister), Lynch began to write out instructions for his own—again. He had, he said, been drawing up his funeral plans since he was at least twenty: as an "exercise in management" or "exercise in confrontation." But *"as the real thing grows closer—next year? 2010?—I find a growing impatience with the entertainment. I'd prefer postponing such a service as long as possible. I want treatments, now."* To the extent that he did envision a service, Lynch said that he would want an "utterly secular" funeral, with *"none of this nonsense about 'we are here to celebrate life.'"* Anyone who wanted that *"should go to a birthday party or a disco with a damned good DJ."*

Throughout August, Lynch continued to suffer from lack of energy and was frustrated when his doctor could find nothing wrong and pronounced him to be fine. But at the beginning of September he was diagnosed with his first opportunistic infection, PCP, and wondered if that meant he *"might have a little adjustment to make in leaving public life for the fall."* Lynch made every effort to stay at home, but two weeks later, on September 14, he was admitted to the Toronto General Hospital. *"If this thing explodes,"* he thought—with the experience of Bill Lewis and Ray Gray in mind—he would feel a sense of urgency about taking care of his latest project, setting up the Toronto Centre for Gay and Lesbian Studies; and he would feel *"grief at not advancing with the book, and of course an oceanic regret at leaving a life and a son I love with such pleasure."* But nine days later, after a hospital stay prolonged because of an adverse reaction to intravenous pentamidine, Lynch returned home.

He was discouraged, and the death of forty-four-year-old Alan Dewar less than two weeks later did not help. *"Alan was a fiery, combative, no-nonsense force in forming AAN!"* he wrote. Dewar had been instrumental in setting up the Community Initiative for AIDS Research in Toronto, and was a director of that body when he died.[3]

Lynch was now detached from AAN! and feeling glad about that. He noted that George Smith had tried to draw him back in. *"But I think now (at a distance) what I thought (while in the thick): it's not very successful. We haven't mobilized and the governments are as terrible on AIDS as ever."* Although he had been the prime mover behind the formation of the organization, Lynch didn't even attend AAN!'s first annual general meeting on October 5th.

What energy he had—he was on sick leave from the university during the fall—went to other projects. For example, a big event in his life was the first meeting, on November 25, of the board of the Toronto Centre for Lesbian and Gay Studies, another of his ambitious undertakings. The Centre would be committed to fostering lesbian and gay studies—both academic and community-based—

throughout the country, with a particular focus on Canadian, historical, and minority studies.[4] Lynch outlined its purpose:

> We want to highlight the diversity of activity and study already available in the community. We also want to be a catalyst for encouraging further work to fill the many gaps in our knowledge and analysis. The Centre Board fully endorses the principle that people of colour should be empowered to speak for themselves and from the perspective of their culture.[5]

Despite Lynch's apparent disappointment with the organization, AAN! was successfully drawing attention to critical issues around treatment and care for people with HIV/AIDS. In mid-September AAN! called for an end to Fisons' aerosolized pentamidine trial using placebos, noting that more than thirty leading U.S. researchers, doctors, civil libertarians, and journalists had signed a statement declaring that Canadian trials be stopped.[6] In addition to staging demonstrations, AAN! members were also working behind the scenes, meeting with politicians and government bureaucrats. In the summer, George Smith, Chuck Grochmal, and Dr. Michael Hulton met with Dr. R.M. MacMillan, Ontario's assistant deputy minister for the community health division, and provincial AIDS co-ordinator Dr. Evelyn Wallace. Afterwards Smith wrote to them, first applauding the province's decision to convene a consensus conference on AIDS, which had been a key demand of AAN! from its first public meeting. (The Working Conference on AIDS and HIV would be held December 1–2, 1989. It was limited to 140 volunteer participants representing professions and organizations actively providing services for people with HIV/AIDS or monitoring the disease.)[7] Smith urged the Ministry of Health to prepare for that conference by commissioning a "baseline" report on the state of delivery of medical services to people with HIV/AIDS. He warned of "a rising tide of anger" in Toronto over the failure of the medical profession, hospitals, and the government to provide leadership and innovative management strategies for the delivery of health services. "People afflicted with AIDS require more than palliative care," Smith wrote. "Public health announcements extolling the virtues of condoms have come too late for them. They expect state-of-the-art treatment for their disease, and have every right to it."[8]

At the annual general meeting in October, AAN! members adopted seven main policies that, if acted on, would add up to better treatment and care for people with HIV/AIDS. One of the key demands was for recognition of the role of "catastrophic rights"—understood, essentially, as the unrestricted right of access by people with HIV/AIDS and others in life-threatening situations to treatments that they and their physicians believed to be beneficial. The treatments should be available free of charge, even if they did not have government approval for regular distribution.[9] As AAN! stated: "Our government continues to deny us treatments that have proven successful elsewhere and in collusion with the pharmaceutical industry is inflicting unethical placebo testing on Canadians in life threatening situations." Secondly, AAN! reiterated its stand against placebo testing, but added that it "supports full testing of drugs"—stipulating that the drugs should be available in catastrophic situations even while they were still undergoing tests and that the tests could be done using either historical or comparative controls. The five other policies demanded that anonymous testing be made widely available, that all boards and committees dealing with people with HIV/AIDS should have some of those people as members, that a national treatment registry be established, that standard protocols be established for hospitals (instead of a "hit and miss" approach to AIDS care), and that a comprehensive approach to home care be developed.[10] In the spring of 1990 AAN! did set up its own treatment information exchange, which by February 1991 had evolved into an independent charitable organization, the Community AIDS Treatment Information Exchange (CATIE).

In its early days, AAN! was loosely organized. "Meetings were held in people's houses, and they went on forever," Brent Southin recalled. "Then we started meeting at the 519 Community Centre, where you can only rent rooms for two hours at a time." As chair McCaskell was excellent at running a tight meeting, Southin said.

There was, according to McCaskell, no criticism of Lynch's gradual withdrawal from AAN! "Michael wasn't very well . . . nobody said, where's Michael? He ended up doing other stuff. I think people start criticizing each other when organizations are in real trouble. At that point, AAN! was still in a period of formation, and there was lots of momentum, things were moving along."

Glen Brown recalled that some AAN! members were "astonished" to see Lynch spearheading the AIDS Memorial. "A number of us were very wary of any talk about mourning because it sounded like those old days when that was all there was. What did it have to do with activism? So again, Michael helped to bridge the gap." Lynch would, "very gently," argue that mourning and activism were not opposite and that, indeed, if they were both done properly they could fuel one another. Mourning meant remembering what the community had learned and could learn from the person being mourned. But more, it also meant remembering how difficult it was to mourn—which meant that the community should do everything it possibly could to stop having to mourn more people, which in turn meant taking action.

Clinical trials and terrors of resurrection

In mid-November 1988 AAN! members travelled to London, Ontario, to present the activist point of view to participants at the first-ever Conference on Clinical Trials in HIV Disease in Canada. There were demonstrators outside the conference, and a few activists attended the meetings. Dr. Philip Berger, who went to the conference as a Toronto doctor with a large AIDS practice, said his most vivid memory of the event was of Chuck Grochmal standing up in front of the participants, calmly but firmly putting his fist down on a table and warning the assembled doctors, researchers, drug company representatives, and government functionaries, "We can shut down any clinical trial in this country."

Grochmal was "so resolute," Berger recalled. "He spoke in a calm, deliberate, and unambiguous way. The room froze. That was a turning point."

Never before had a "patient group" collectively recognized their own power within the research setting in Canada. Never before had a group of research subjects threatened to so directly unbalance the process of scientific research. "That was the power that smartened people up," recalls Dr. Michele Brill-Edwards, who also remembered Grochmal's warning. She attended the meeting in her position as a representative of the Health Protection Branch's Bureau of Human Prescription Drugs. The activists had legitimate rights. They were saying, "If you won't play ball with us, we won't play ball with you. We won't enter your clinical trials, or we'll enter placebo trials and we'll share pills." According to Brill-Edwards, both the researchers and the drug companies got the message. "If patients shared pills, the trial wouldn't show any difference between the two groups, and drug companies ran the risk of being worse off if they submitted the results for drug approval." The drug trials would become ungovernable if catastrophic rights were not recognized.

Persuaded by activists, researchers at the London conference agreed that, during trials of promising AIDS drugs, HIV-positive patients who didn't want to enrol in a trial and run the risk of receiving a placebo would be given access to trial drugs through a third, open treatment arm of the trial. (This idea was similar to a proposal for a "parallel track" for investigational AIDS drugs put forward by ACT UP in the United States. In June 1989 Anthony Fauci of the National Institute of Allergy and Infectious Diseases endorsed the "parallel track.")[11] AAN! had argued that a placebo-controlled trial is only ethical "when research and treatment are completely divorced." Subjects must enter placebo-controlled drug trials with the view of contributing to science, and not as the only way of getting treatment for their illness or disease."[12] This was also the view of the Medical Research Council of Canada, but as AAN! discovered, precious few researchers and bureaucrats seemed aware of it. AAN! chair McCaskell was quick to write to the doctor in change of an upcoming double-blind placebo trial of the drug Ribavirin, reminding her of the London decision to offer an open-treatment arm.[13]

In early December, Lynch was excited by reports of a passive immunotherapy technique being experimented with in England. *"Haven't been so gung-ho for a therapy since AZT . . . But will it be two years before it's tried here?"* The technique involved taking plasma from asymptomatic people, treating it for viral and bacterial infection, and injecting it into HIV-positive people with low levels of AIDS-fighting cells. The theory was that asymptomatic HIV-positive people have high antibody levels (titres) and that AIDS patents have lower levels, and that perhaps the antibodies are protective. AAN! invited Dr. Abram Karpas, the British veterinarian who was experimenting with the approach, to speak in Toronto.[14]

Lynch had been a regular at the Modern Language Association (MLA) meetings held every year during the Christmas break, but did not feel up to attending the convention in New Orleans at the end of 1988. He was still fatigued and continued to have night sweats, which he ranked in terms of the number of T-shirt changes required: light, one change; medium, two or three changes; heavy, four or five changes. Instead, he sent a paper, "Terrors of Resurrection," which Eve Kosofsky Sedgwick presented on his behalf. The paper was about perceptions of AIDS, and it was nominally related to his discipline of English Literature. It opened, for example, by referring to a poem he had written in the mid-1970s. He wrote the paper, he said, "in a lit crit mode," but the key issue—the question of strong resistance to the AIDS = Death "frame"—came out of AIDS Action Now!

"Terrors of Resurrection" examined the general resistance to accepting the reality that AIDS was becoming a chronic, manageable disease like diabetes. Advances in clinical care had taken place, including not only approaches to prevent the opportunistic infections that had proved fatal in the past but also strategies of early intervention. But despite those advances, "AIDS is so firmly ligatured to death, in our framing of it, and to apocalypse, that we cannot easily locate alternatives," Lynch argued. Meanwhile, resistance to a new way of thinking about AIDS was prevalent both among groups like the Moral Majority in the United States and in "the doers of good, often genuine good, who overcome their distaste for marginalized sexuality or even marginalized drug use *as long as the marginalized are safely dying away*." He added:

> Resistance occurs in medical workers, social workers, families of diagnosed: how much we love you, how much we want to do for you, since you are dying. Resistance is most firmly entrenched in the media, where boilerplate lines such as "nearly always fatal" mar even stories about improved treatment prospects. Resistance also occurs in people who accept their positive antibody test as a sentence to death.[15]

Lynch's argument resonates a full decade and a half later. What seems curious is that he picked an academic setting to outline his thoughts—or, at least, that he didn't rework his ideas in an article for a publication that would reach a wider audience.

Sadness and frustration

As 1989 began, Lynch was happy to be back teaching after his sick leave. He was also informed that the MLA gay caucus, in which he'd been very active, had established an award in his name. According to his friend Linda Hutcheon, a University of Toronto professor, an award like that, in someone's name, "is not standard. It was a mark of the impact he had made on the gay scholarly community."[16]

But the deaths and illnesses continued. Ken Calendar, a friend from his New York circle, died on January 5. A couple of weeks later Craig Liske, a fellow undergraduate at Oberlin College, died of AIDS contracted from a blood transfusion during surgery. In Toronto there was an AIDS death and partner suicide of Lynch's acquaintances (Bob Metcalfe and Jacques Aubin-Roy). His friend Gram Campbell was diagnosed with his third bout of PCP, and Jacques D'Angenais, who had designed the AIDS Memorial, was hospitalized.

From Los Angeles, on the occasion of Calendar's death, Bruce Schentes wrote a joint letter to Lynch, Spiers, and Michael Jorgensen:

> I want to be with you guys right now. It isn't right that Herb should have to deal with Ken's death without the physical presence/presents of the old family. It was the one thing I often thought about when Dr. C and I started our exodus from Gotham. Indeed, the week we left I suspected we would be returning to Ken's bedside not too long after to say goodbye. Ken fooled us, didn't he? Instead, there were a few phone calls. They were distant more in their content than their actuality. It was as if Ken had already said his goodbyes to us and I felt as if we were imposing on his self-isolation. We stopped calling, relied on your status reports, and put him in that special place already occupied by the rest we love and can no longer share day to day stuff.
>
> When Herb called to tell us Ken had died, I heard myself thinking, "Of course he died. He died last year. What's he doing dying again? I don't want to grieve again." And I didn't. I didn't cry.

I didn't feel the loss. I did/do feel guilty. Ken deserves all that feeling his sisters brought up. I don't know, it seems that just when you think you've got it down, they change the rules on you.

All these months I had just assumed that I'd be joining all of you to say goodbye to Ken and when the time came it didn't seem right. And yet it doesn't seem right that I'm not there either.

I miss the "family." Pines summers and dinners at the loft seem closer in time than whatever it was I did last week. I still imagine camping with Steve, gossiping with Blair, and dreaming with Ray as if they were here right now. When I entered your lives and you mine ten years ago, I brought with me all the naivete that a kid from Kansas was expected to bring. You all taught me about love and friendship and relationships and how to enjoy life—all those things that have kept me going during the shit. It was Ken and Blair who made the introduction.

I can't/shouldn't complain—but I will. I'm very lucky. I have David, and 3,000 miles will never separate me from my Herb and my Michaels. But I wish we were drinking champagne and eating nachos on the 8th floor tonight [at Ray Gray's studio apartment in Herb's building]. We have good friends out here, but it's not the same. I keep looking for something; trying to get it all back. Maybe it's because our biggest concern 10 years ago was our next dinner, next party, next dance, next drug. Maybe it's because you were all my mentors in many respects. Maybe it's because I'm ten years older. But I can't find a family that gives me all the good stuff and bad . . .

I feel more than slightly relieved that Ken is now dancing with the girls rather than watching game shows in bed. And what keeps me from being afraid of low t cells and rashes is knowing that there is a dance going on somewhere. I also know that the music will still be playing whenever I get there, so I'll stick around for a while, watch the niece and nephew grow up, throw a few frisbees and hope that you, me, and those we can hold now can dance at least one more dance down here together.

I miss you guys. And love you more than I'm sure I've ever told you.

Bruce (Tessa de la Swamp)[17]

In Canada frustration with the federal government's inaction on AIDS was mounting. On January 16, 1989, *The Toronto Star* ran a story quoting Tak Mak slamming the government. An internationally renowned Canadian virologist and immunologist who had contributed to the landmark 1988 Royal Society of Canada report on AIDS, Mak was not known for speaking to the press. "There is no concerted effort, no leadership, no vision and no plan to fight against AIDS in Canada," he told Kelly Toughill, the newspaper's AIDS reporter. "We have the second highest AIDS rate in the industrialized world, but we aren't doing anything about it. . . . We are going to have to wait until people close to the government start getting AIDS before we see concerted action."[18]

Ernest McCulloch, president of the Academy of Sciences, the scientific arm of the Royal Society, told the *Star*: "The government pressured us when we were conducting the study to move more rapidly. They gave us every indication that they approved of the recommendations, but then they put the report on the shelf." Dr. Philip Berger charged that the government was "dabbling around as if the disease started yesterday. If the bureaucrats were forced just once to sit across a table and tell a patient he's infected, they might stop dragging their heels."[19]

The drug debacle

But things were about to change, thanks to the hard work of AIDS activists and a widely viewed CBC-Television item, "The Nassau Connection," which first aired on the program *Monitor* on January 16, 1989. The program was about Dextran Sulphate, the experimental AIDS treatment that Lynch had, in the spring of 1988, managed to obtain through San Francisco/Japan connections. "The Nassau Connection" exposed the bureaucratic mess that was so frustrating to AIDS patients and their doctors. Dextran Sulphate had been used in Japan for twenty years to treat high cholesterol, and in 1987 Japanese researchers had reported in *The Lancet* on evidence that the drug could halt replication of the AIDS virus. A major producer of the substance was a firm called Polydex, located in Scarborough in Metropolitan Toronto. But the drug had not gone through clinical trials, and the federal government's Health Protection Branch refused to permit its sale in Canada. Instead the Canadian-manufactured drug was available in Nassau, Bahamas, and AIDS activists were buying it from there and having it shipped north. This route sidestepped the regulatory issue, since Health Canada allowed patients to import small quantities of experimental drugs for personal use. The *Monitor* program featured David Marriage, a PWA with advanced Kaposi's sarcoma who had succeeded in obtaining the drug from Nassau. Marriage described the toll that the endeavour was taking on him and Grochmal, who was trying to obtain an affordable supply anywhere he could through buyers' clubs set up by PWAS.

Federal officials flatly contradicted each other on camera and provided misleading information. Alastair Clayton, head of the Federal Centre for AIDS, insisted that the drug was not and should not be available until it had been tested to be safe. Then he said the drug would be available under the Emergency Drug Release Program (EDRP), "when it is in Canada." When the interviewer pointed out that the drug already was in Canada, Clayton replied that the pills "had not been submitted to the system."

In 1987–88 the Emergency Drug Release Program had approved 7,515 emergency drug releases, according to a federal document, but until January 1989 it appeared that none of those releases had included drugs to treat AIDS or AIDS-related conditions.[20] The mandate of the EDRP, according to a 1981 medical journal article, was to authorize the sale of drugs to a doctor for a specified patient "when a medical emergency exists and standard therapy is not effective. . . . Most requests are handled by the directorate very promptly, and most North American pharmaceutical companies ship the drugs rapidly within 24 hours."[21] The EDRP was routinely used by various divisions within the Health Protection Branch to release, for example, experimental cardiovascular drugs, and experimental cancer drugs. A 1988 federal document noted that drugs typically released through the EDRP included orphan drugs "for which the demand in Canada is so small that it would never be profitable for a company to market them" and "drug products for which no manufacturer has yet submitted an NDS [New Drug Submission]." (Pentamidine had been granted "orphan drug status" in the United States, where it was widely used in an aerosolized form, an "off-label" use.)[22]

On "The Nassau Connection," Mary Carman Kasparek, chief of the drug regulatory affairs section of the Health Protection Branch, told interviewers that Dextran Sulphate could be obtained within twenty-four hours through the EDRP by calling a twenty-four-hour hotline. She said there had been no requests for Dextran Sulphate through the EDRP. She also "warned" that the drug caused diarrhea, which will "kill AIDS patients faster," at which point the program cut away to Marriage, who responded, "I'm sorry, I have AIDS . . . my life is at stake."

When Dr. Michael Hulton, Grochmal's physician, telephoned the EDRP hotline in Ottawa—at the urging of the television interviewers and on camera—to apply for the drug, he was told in no uncertain terms that the drug was not available and that Kasparek had no business telling him it would be.[23]

According to Brill-Edwards, who by December 1, 1988, had been appointed assistant deputy minister of the Bureau of Infectious Diseases in the Health Protection Branch, when "The Nassau Connection" first aired the program caused some internal discomfort in Ottawa. The first broadcast was restricted to Southern Ontario. But when the program was rebroadcast nationally eight days later on *The Journal*, the newsmagazine program that ran after the CBC nightly national news, it caused "an explosion like a firestorm," Brill-Edwards said. The day after the program aired nationally, Brill-Edwards was put in charge of the portfolio. She acted immediately to implement the EDRP. "To me, the patients had a legitimate claim," she said later. "It's like the angry relatives of someone who is ill—in medicine you treat them well, because they have good reason to be angry. Whereas the bureaucratic imperative is to argue and deny. It seemed to me we had to proceed." Eager to avoid further embarrassment, the politicians and bureaucrats backed up the move. Within days, Health and Welfare Canada decided to make both aerosolized pentamidine and Dextran Sulphate available through the EDRP.[24]

The Dextran Sulphate debacle, especially since the drug was manufactured in Canada, best revealed the "absurdity" of the situation—a point that Tim McCaskell made on the television program. But the release of aerosolized pentamidine through the EDRP was far more important to people with AIDS, because its efficacy was already clear and PCP was a leading cause of death among people with AIDS. AAN! had been operating its own Pentamidine Project for nine months, obtaining the drug from the United States so that close to one hundred PWAS had access to aerosolized pentamidine. Within four months of the decision by the federal government, Ontario announced that it was setting up its own aerosolized pentamidine clinic at a medical clinic in downtown Toronto, predicting that up to one thousand people a year would use the facility.[25]

Soon after those drugs were released, a host of other experimental drugs were made available through the EDRP. By February the list of experimental drugs to be made available "on compassionate grounds" through the EDRP for AIDS was expanded to also include AZT, EL10 (DHEA), and, for AIDS-related illnesses, Gancyclovir, alpha-interferon, and a host of others.[26]

The decision to release aerosolized pentamidine and Dextran Sulphate in January 1989 was not a new policy, but a matter of enforcing an old one, Brill-Edwards told *The Toronto Star*.[27] Years later Brill-Edwards said that, in retrospect, she attributed the previous non-release of AIDS drugs through the EDRP to the domination of the infectious disease directorate by scientists, rather than medical doctors. "They seemed to feel it was their job to be the guardian of drugs and not let doctors have access. They'd say AZT was a toxin. I'd say so are most [experimental] cancer drugs." For other drugs released under EDRP, the Health Protection Branch allowed for the potential of a huge ADR (Adverse Drug Reaction). Indeed, Brill-Edwards said she was surprised that no one took legal action against the government given that, before 1989, the EDRP had not been properly administered in the infectious diseases division. "To my amazement and relief, the press and patients did not come back at us. They could have sued the pants off us."

The availability of drugs through the EDRP did not immediately help patients. Brill-Edwards returned to her office early in the spring to find staff in a panic. Activists in Vancouver had announced that they were planning a mass demonstration to embarrass Health Minister Perrin Beatty during a scheduled visit to the city. She telephoned Greig Layne of the Vancouver PWA Coalition, who explained the issue to her. Aerosolized pentamidine was now available through the EDRP, but doctors weren't applying under the program because they didn't know that it worked. They had no information on it. Drug companies would normally only supply information after a drug went to market, and not before. By this time, Lyphomed—a U.S. competitor of Fisons, which was running the placebo trial in Canada—had reported its own findings to the U.S. Food and Drug Administration (FDA) based on trials that it had helped sponsor. Lyphomed had worked with the AIDS community and ran trials comparing different doses of aerosolized pentamidine, instead of placebos. The trials were conducted at both the Community Research Initiative in New York and San Francisco's County Community Consortium of Bay Area HIV Health Care Providers. According to Brill-Edwards, these tests did result in information that could be shared with the doctors, but because the drug had not been approved, the company could not make any announcements or share any findings.

Brill-Edwards proposed that Health Canada's Health Protection Branch issue a letter to doctors, stating that studies submitted to the FDA had demonstrated the efficacy of aerosolized pentamidine. "The deputy minister said, do what it takes." A letter was written the next day (although it took much longer for final bureaucratic approval), and the Vancouver demonstration was averted.[28] By the end of 1989, a special AIDS division had been created within the Bureau of Infectious Diseases.

Poetry: a thing with feathers

A month or two into 1989, Lynch's opinion of AAN!'s achievements had improved. About a demonstration at Toronto's Don Jail, he wrote: *"I went out of duty but it was so **good** (good goals, clear strategies, large gathering) I had a good time."*[29] AAN! had set up a committee concerned with the rights of prisoners with AIDS. That same day Spiers called from New York to report another two deaths among their friends: Don Ott and Tom Stehling.

The next month was largely taken up with travel and socializing, as Lynch launched his new book of poetry, *These Waves of Dying Friends*, in New York, San Francisco, and Toronto. In New York, after a reading at A Different Light bookstore, he hosted a small reception attended by local luminaries like historian George Chauncey and literary theorist Kate Stimpson, and did not stint on the refreshments (he paid $134 U.S. for one of the bottles of wine). In San Francisco his reading was attended by a crowd including Allan Bérubé, David Miller, and Pat Bond. When he was halfway through reading his poem "Yellow Kitchen Gloves" at that launch, his copy of the book ran out of pages—and it turned out that all of the copies at the bookstore were missing half their pages. At the Toronto launch, held on March 3 at an art gallery on Spadina Avenue, Scott Cline told Lynch that he had been reacting to the epidemic "by rejecting all the pleasure in our disco years. You made me remember how much fun we had." After another Toronto reading, at Glad Day Bookshop, Lynch dropped into the hospital to visit D'Angenais, who had already received last rites. When Lynch finally arrived home, he found Othello, the cat he had inherited from Lewis, stretched out and stiff from rigor mortis at the foot of his bed. He took the cat's body to the veterinarian for cremation and *"walked away without Othello in my hands, in my care. I felt light, unburdened, & alone and it was then, walking down Davenport towards Bay, I cried. Now the house seems very empty. My left arm wants to reach out and stroke him as I write, in our favourite bed position."*

Lynch received a fundraising letter from the Family Practice Unit of the Toronto General Hospital, where he had been a patient in the fall. He promptly shipped the letter back with a handwritten comment: "When TGH stops marking AIDS patients' rooms with 'Enteric Blood Precaution' signs, and adopts (as Women's College has) *universal precautions,* I will consider a donation. But not with this current offensive policy." After a few weeks the doctor in charge of the unit replied: "Our current policy of labelling certain patients' room for special precautions is not only offensive, as you point out, but also has been shown to be ineffective when compared to a universal precautions policy. Because of this, the hospital is moving to abandon this specific labelling and adoption of universal body substance precautions. However, as often happens in an institution of this size, progress is dishearteningly slow."[30] While large teaching hospitals adopted universal precautions, the custom of identifying the rooms of AIDS patients with special hazard signs persisted for years in some smaller hospitals.

In April Lynch became completely immersed in Wagner's "Ring Cycle," and at the end of the month went with his friend Gerald Hannon to the Metropolitan Opera in New York to see it performed. Meanwhile, he was heartened by reports of another new AIDS treatment being investigated in San Francisco: *"My mind begins to toy with the idea of a lifespan carrying me **past** 50 or 51. What a readjustment to make! A thing with feathers."* Lynch had, for several months, been experiencing bouts of lack of bowel control. On one occasion he cleaned up but forgot to change his underwear. He went off to a birthday party with *"a hint of the outhouse about me."*

Chaos, the blues, and a conference

In mid-April 1989 Dr. Norbert Gilmore, the respected chairman of the National Advisory Committee on AIDS, resigned his position. Gilmore, who had headed the Committee since 1983, publicly declared that Canada's program to fight AIDS was a mess. His comments corroborated the criticism that AIDS activists had long been levelling at the government. "For years we have been living on the promise that something would be done tomorrow," Gilmore said. "Well, these people have been at it for more than six years now and we still don't have the programs that we need . . . it's chaos."[31] More than 2,500 Canadians had been diagnosed with AIDS, and experts estimated that up to 50,000 were infected with HIV. But Canada, unlike most other industrialized nations, had no national strategy to combat the epidemic. Gilmore said the federal government was fast off the mark to keep track of AIDS cases, but slammed it for inaction on education to prevent AIDS. He saved his greatest criticism for how the government had handled the issue of drugs. The worst failing had been in the area of experimental drugs, because the government had not sponsored clinical trials of promising drugs or developed a policy on access to experimental drugs.

In a paper delivered the following October, Gilmore gave credit to the AIDS community for its activism on drugs. Community development had led, he said, "to an extensive information network about therapeutic interventions, to high-profile consumer advocacy, and to an 'underground' marketplace for these agents." The community had increased its participation in both the design of clinical trials and their conduct. "Without community participation and support, much of what is known about the HIV epidemic and its treatment would now be unknown," Gilmore said. Still, despite all the participation, data on drug trials—on what affected recruitment into, and compliance with, them—was limited.[32]

In Gilmore's view, part of the battle over AIDS had been lost back in 1984–85, when the Health Protection Branch, with its "contain and control" attitude, was vying for new dollars with a Health Promotion Branch, whose approach was more participatory. According to Gilmore, the Health Protection Branch won, and the National Advisory Council on AIDS was gradually "strangled."

Perrin Beatty replaced Jake Epp as federal minister of health and shortly afterwards, on May 9, 1989, the new minister acknowledged some of the government's failings. "I would have liked to have seen a national [AIDS] strategy in place well before now," he told *The Medical Post*.[33] But instead, Beatty said, he had inherited "a legacy of poor communications with the key players in the AIDS battle." Meanwhile, Beatty made no promise to have an AIDS strategy in place quickly. On the advice of AIDS groups, he said, he was going to consult extensively before formulating such a strategy.

Seemingly far from those concerns, in mid-May Lynch began teaching a summer course on effective writing and planting his back garden entirely in blue plants and flowers, *"in part to resonate with Bessie [Smith] and Billie [Holiday] and my foster home: the blues."* After attending a play based on Malcolm X's break from Elijah Mohammed, Lynch pondered:

> *Why do I feel comfortable these days only w/black or other minorities' cultural material—in which, of course, I'm a tourist only? One thing is that it's an edge, as I've always felt better at the edge. The institutionalization of gay studies is happening so fast, and entrenching such lily-white careerist conservatism, I feel truly sidelined by it.*

For him, the Michael Lynch Award established by the MLA gay caucus meant that he was now considered to be *"superannuated, 'loved,' safe, and useless."* Now he felt himself wanting *"to be useful as an anti-racist, and a challenger of cracker hegemony."* The Toronto Centre for Lesbian and Gay Studies that he had helped to set up was not in great shape, he thought, *"and that's largely because I don't know how to lead it, or where. How to be community-based w/o being anti-intellectual?"*

For months AAN! and ACT UP had been preparing for the Fifth International Conference on AIDS, to be held in Montreal in June 1989. The conference would be the largest gathering of researchers to discuss one disease in the history of science: 11,600 researchers with 5,302 new studies in their book of abstracts. It was also the second conference in a row in which the U.S. government had no major test results to report from any large-scale drug studies. The most dramatic breakthrough discussed was aerosolized pentamidine, now that its efficacy had been proved by community doctors in San Francisco.[34] The drug was formally approved by the U.S. Food and Drug Administration on June 15, 1989.

Activists had not had much say or presence at the Fourth international AIDS conference in Stockholm in 1988. The annual conferences had become a platform for the AIDS industry—medical experts, government bureaucrats, and pharmaceutical companies— and activists in both Canada and the United States were determined that Montreal would be different. George Smith observed that more and more AIDS organizations across Canada were becoming activist-oriented "because of the new treatments and the possibility of PWAS surviving."[35] ACT UP, meanwhile, decided that the conference presented "an ideal opportunity to bring our message to a worldwide audience . . . if this conference sets the tone for the way that AIDS will be handled for the next year, we want to make it an activists' agenda."[36] Thanks to pressure from the Canadian AIDS Society, a person with HIV/AIDS had been appointed to the conference planning committee. CAS had also fought successfully for an agenda that included involvement by people with AIDS.

ACT UP and AAN! worked together to produce the Montreal Manifesto, also known as "The Declaration of the Universal Rights and Needs of People Living with HIV Disease." On May 22, Herb

Spiers sent a revised copy of the manifesto from New York to Chuck Grochmal in Toronto. In a covering letter, he noted that the document was to go to ACT UP's co-ordinating committee in a few days: "I hope that AAN! is prepared to release this on its own if there are unanticipated problems here." Glen Brown had been chosen to liaise with ACT UP, and travelled to New York to talk with Spiers. "They were New York ACT UP and they weren't used to working in coalition on an equal footing," Brown said later. "But given that, I think we did fairly well." The Montreal Manifesto made ten demands on behalf of people with HIV/AIDS worldwide, including a call for governments to ensure access and availability of treatments, a code of rights for people with HIV/AIDS, an international data bank to share all medical information related to the syndrome, culturally sensitive international education programs, and an international development fund to assist poor countries in meeting their health-care responsibilities. (Almost all of the demands remain today as unmet needs.)

AAN! members were scheduled to arrive in Montreal on June 2 to set up an "action centre," working with Réaction-SIDA (Syndrome d'immuno déficience acquise), a small Montreal-based activist group. (Réaction-SIDA, which included many Anglophone as well as Francophone gay men, had coalesced in the period leading up to the conference but did not survive long after it.) Stefan Lynch had registered for the conference to learn more about AIDS, and was also determined to take part in any activism. As a computer-savvy young man, Stefan was impressed with the action centre. About half the activists attending the conference were admitted with forged passes, he said. "They had computers and laser printers and they were just churning these things out. There were press passes. It was, in my consciousness, the first sort of high-tech protest of the information age, although it really wasn't since it wasn't organized on the net . . . But to my seventeen-year-old mind, it was like they're on it, this is cool."

The Canadian AIDS Society was meeting in Montreal (June 2 to 4), just prior to the international conference, and AAN! chair Tim McCaskell had been invited to facilitate a workshop on AIDS activism and discuss plans for activism during the conference. One day before the conference began, AAN! stalwart Bernard Courte was hired by the International Development Research Council, which was cosponsoring the conference, to work as a media liaison officer with representatives of the gay press. It was the first time there had been such a position at an international AIDS conference. Courte had been involved with AAN! since 1988 and had created its Francophone section; from early on AIDS *Action News!* had articles in both English and French.

Absent from the AAN! or ACT UP planning documents was any mention of the central action at the conference. ACT UP, AAN! and Réaction-SIDA had been holding joint planning meetings, and the official plan for the opening ceremony was, essentially, "to march around outside and yell and scream" to make their point, Brown said. Instead, without informing AAN! members, a contingent of ACT UP demonstrators started to lead the group *inside* the convention centre to take over the opening ceremonies. That was how ACT UP operated. "They didn't call it a cell," Brown explained, "but they had a SWAT team and they would design an action and not everyone was told because if they knew, they wouldn't agree." McCaskell and Brown were lead marshals for the demonstration, and when the ACT UP strategy became obvious they decided to get in front and take the lead. Not telling the Canadians about the plan was a mistake, said Spiers, who had known about it in advance. "Though when it did happen, they were quick to respond."

Demonstrators swept into the Palais des Congrès, riding up the escalators to the main convention hall while chanting "The whole world is watching" and waving placards—"Silence = Death" and "The world is sick of government genocide."[37] "You just felt like you were rising up into this space and taking control," Stefan said. "There was a sense that this is now our space, and it rightfully belongs to us because no one is more affected." The group went onto the stage and took over the podium without so much as a scuffle. "People were waiting for the speakers to start, and we took it over, chanting," Stefan said. "A couple of hundred of us around the podium and on the floor."

AAN!'s McCaskell grabbed the microphone. "On behalf of people living with AIDS in Canada and around the world, I would like to officially open the Fifth International Conference on AIDS," he declared. McCaskell upstaged Canadian Prime Minister Brian Mulroney, who was to open the conference officially with an address that would mark his first-ever public remarks on AIDS—after having been prime minister for five years.[38] McCaskell told the conference that Mulroney's remarks would constitute "an unprecedented historical piece of political hypocrisy given the record of the Mulroney government on AIDS." The government, he said, "has totally failed to plan or provide treatment for an epidemic that is now nine years old."[39] The Montreal Manifesto was read aloud in English and French. "We were shouting and screaming and the researchers [in the audience] had no context," said Stefan. "There had been big ACT UP protests in the United States, but mostly about bureaucratic processes, not scientific ones." The researchers were interested in what was going on. "It was a spectacle," Stefan said. "They did not get the sense that it was a threat."

After more than an hour, the protestors left the stage and took seats among the other audience members. "There was this funny moment of you are us, and we are you . . . that line between witness and protestor rarely gets broken," Stefan said. There had been no great confrontation or struggle. There was not necessarily a division between activists and scientists, and many doctors had been politicized by the problems around access to drugs and the lack of appropriate federal funding. Stefan was left there, sitting amongst these strangers, feeling somewhat uncomfortable and tense. Greig Layne of Vancouver thought that most of the conference participants welcomed the activists and embraced them as allies. "The only people on the opposite side of the fence were the drug companies and the politicians, as usual."[40] Kevin Brown, the crusading activist from Vancouver, was to have addressed the opening session of the conference, but Brown had died of AIDS on May 9. A video compilation of interviews with him was shown on huge screens in the main convention hall.

When Mulroney came to the podium and began to speak, the activists in the audience, including Stefan, stood up and turned their backs on him.[41] They undid their wrist watches and, silently, held them up. The audience quickly realized what was happening with the activists standing facing them, with their wrist watches in the air, especially when someone shouted out, "It's been nine years, why haven't you said anything before!"

"For me it was an amazing moment," said Stefan. "First of all it was really cathartic, because here was the one person it was easiest to be angry at." It was all about societal taboos and inaction, he said, about frustration and anger. "It is nine years into the epidemic and this is the first time you are saying the word AIDS! Why had Bill died? Why is my Dad sick? And you've done nothing!" Stefan said he suffered some discomfort, being stared at by the crowd, but even with a thousand eyes staring at him he had a firm sense of justification. "I am outraged and I am justified and I am going to keep standing here," he thought. At age seventeen, still not able to vote, not yet able to participate fully in politics, he found himself engaged in an extraordinary experience. "I did a lot of AIDS activism after that, but that was the purest, the simplest and the cleanest," he said years later. Stefan was also glad to be there without his father: "The moment of catharsis was mine." Despite the disruption, the next day's *Globe and Mail* managed to report that Mulroney, who had held his ground at the podium, paid "a glowing tribute to Brown and made a moving speech about the civil rights of AIDS patients."[42]

Lynch senior did come to Montreal, but only for one day, to take part in a panel discussion of (once again) "AIDS and the Arts." He told his diary: "*My heart has been heavy, no exaggeration, following news reports of the massacre of students in Bejing. Kent State, to a factor. Mowing down their country people. As these North American governments have let the virus mow us down.*" The Tiananmen Square massacre took place on Sunday, June 4. On June 7, about fifty AIDS activists from the conference joined two thousand people who marched down the streets of Montreal in protest. At the "AIDS and the Arts" panel Lynch spoke of the conflict between his activist politics ("break the AIDS = Death link, give hope") and his efforts to "face down death" in his writing. "*As an activist, I want to give hope . . . when I sit down to write I deal with mortality, mourning, loss. But all mourning is political.*" Indeed, around this time Lynch's poetry was beginning to change, shifting away from the more traditionally elegiac and becoming much more hard-edged.

Returning to Toronto after his panel, Lynch "*came home in a crowded train with shit in my pants.*" Incontinence was still plaguing him.

During the Montreal conference, ACT UP New York released a sixteen-page document, "A National AIDS Treatment Research Agenda." The introduction stated, "Over the last year, dimly, like echoes from a distant battlefield, the voices of people living with AIDS or HIV, and their advocates, have begun to reach the ears of researchers and regulators in the Federal AIDS establishment, who have finally begun to notice that something is wrong." The document called for a comprehensive strategy to address all clinical manifestations of AIDS, outlining twelve principles for a new AIDS drug-testing system. "People with AIDS, HIV and their advocates must participate in designing and executing drug trials" was the first principle. The second was a call for "a comprehensive coordinated compassionate drug development strategy" that would ensure the thorough evaluation of all promising "agents" and, if they were found to be effective, their rapid distribution. The document called for a focus on drugs that would treat or prevent opportunistic infections, not just a focus on antiretroviral drugs, pointing out that there was still no approved treatment for most HIV-related opportunistic infections.[43] ACT UP also called for an end to the exclusion of women, poor people, people in rural areas, people of colour, drug users, prisoners, hemophiliacs, and children from experimental treatments and clinical trials.[44]

The document received little attention from the media, which focused instead on the demonstrations and protests by activists. But some scientists took notice. Susan Ellenberg, chief biostatistician of the U.S. AIDS Clinical Trial Group, said: "I walked down to the courtyard and there was this group of guys, and they were wearing muscle shirts, with earrings and funny hair. I was almost afraid. I was really hesitant even to approach them." But she did, and she read the document and found "many places" where it made sense—where she found herself saying, "You mean, we're not doing this?" or "We're not doing it this way?" After discussions with colleagues, Ellenberg invited representatives from ACT UP and other community-based organizations to participate in her Statistical Working Group.[45]

Two months later AAN! released its own set of policy proposals, "Towards a Comprehensive Federal/Provincial AIDS Policy," with a focused critique of the situation in Canada. The document elaborated on problems within the Federal Centre for AIDS, including its tendency, as a directorate of the Health Protection Branch, to see its mandate purely as a public health function, which kept its interests separate from those of people who were infected with HIV and seeking treatment. "Public health policy and treatment policy in these kinds of catastrophic illnesses are not the same," the document stated. The FCA had seen its mandate as "one of testing the safety and efficacy of proposed AIDS treatments. During its existence it has done absolutely nothing to make new drugs available."[46]

As a result of activism at the conference, Don deGagne of the Vancouver PWA Society was added as a speaker at the closing session, marking the first time a PWA had spoken at the closing of an international AIDS conference. In its evaluation of the conference, AAN! observed that with only about thirty members at the conference, it did not have enough people to accomplish all the necessary tasks. Tripartite facilitation committees of the three activist groups—ACT UP, AAN! and Réaction-SIDA—also did not work well. Better communication between groups and among protestors was vital; and the activists had found themselves unable to control the media agenda. By the time the conference ended, some high-profile personalities, such as Randy Shilts (who gave a closing address), and other conference organizers were trying to construct the activists in their midst as having "gone too far." By that time a number of the activists, especially people from ACT UP, had already left town, and many of those remaining were suffering from exhaustion and not able to respond adequately.

Still, the AAN! document noted that the activists had achieved a significant success in shifting the conference away from being solely an industry platform to ensuring that the needs and concerns of people living with HIV/AIDS were acknowledged: "The enforced invisibility of people living with AIDS at previous international AIDS conferences was ended once and for all." Some activists who had been "feeling rather burnt out were rejuvenated by the activism at the conference."[47]

The document ended with some tentative plans for the Sixth International AIDS conference, to be held in San Francisco in 1990.[48] In the end, though, AIDS activists from around the world boycotted the 1990 conference to protest the U.S. government's official immigration policy, which barred HIV-positive people from admission to the country.

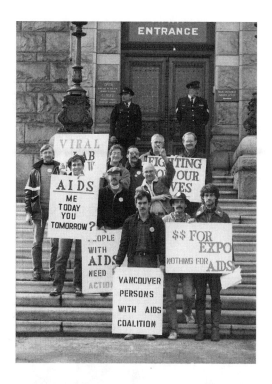

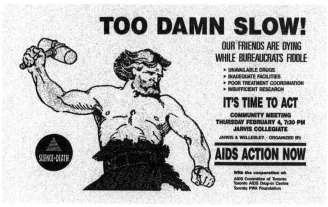

Top: *The first* AIDS *demonstration in Canada: Victoria, B.C., March 26, 1986. The protest at the legislature called for a viral testing lab in the province. Photographer Daniel Collins remembers how nervous everyone was.* Back row from left: *David Pfautz, Warren Jensen (holding sign), unknown, John Kozachenko, Larry [last name unknown], Kevin Brown.* Middle row: *Brian Texiera, Allan Pletcher.* Front: *Unknown, Peter Biggs, Ken Mann.* (Photo: Daniel Collins)

Bottom: Poster designed by Gram Campbell

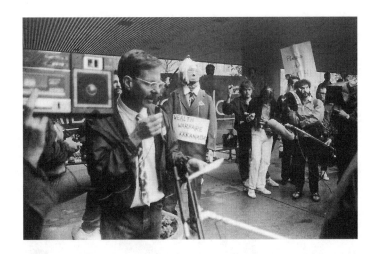

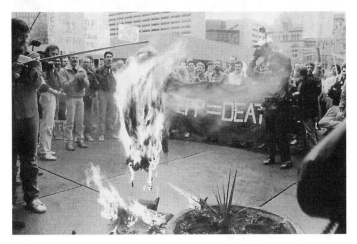

TOP: *Federal Health Minister Jake Epp is "ineducable," Lynch told the crowd at this May 17, 1988, demonstration at Nathan Phillips Square, organized by AIDS Action Now! Protestors at the Toronto demo included participants from the third Canadian Conference on AIDS.* (Photo: Celest Natale)

BOTTOM: *"Fire Epp!" yelled angry protestors as the effigy of Jake Epp, federal minister of health, was consumed with flames. The image captured the attention of the media—and the government—and helped to put AIDS activism firmly on the political agenda.* (Photo: Celest Natale)

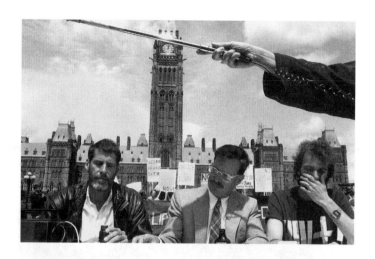

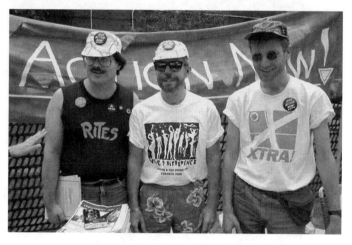

TOP: AIDS *Action Now!* members in front of the Peace Tower on Parliament Hill, taking AIDS *treatments available elsewhere in the world, but not in Canada. Bill Greenway with aerosolized pentamidine, Michael Lynch with Naltrexone, and James Thomas with Dextran Sulphate.* (Photo courtesy of Philip Hannan)

BOTTOM: AIDS *Action Now! stalwarts Gary Kinsman, David Marriage, and Chuck Grochmal hand out literature.* (Photo courtesy of Philip Hannan)

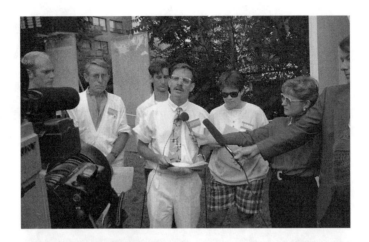

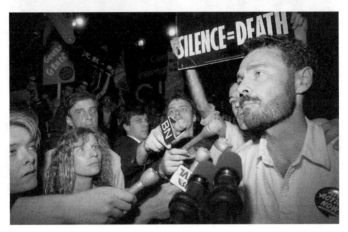

TOP: *Unveiling of the* AIDS *Memorial on Pride Day in Toronto, June 1988. The Memorial was Michael Lynch's brainchild.* (Photo courtesy of Philip Hannan)

BOTTOM: *Activists took over the opening ceremonies of the June 1989 international* AIDS *conference.* AAN! *chair Tim McCaskell, on behalf of people with* AIDS, *declared the conference open.* (Photo courtesy of Philip Hannan)

nine

COMMUNITY STRATEGIES

THE SECOND AIDS MEMORIAL was to open in twelve hours, and Lynch's mood was sombre. *"Deaths this week of David Marriage and Don Briggs have sobered me. Both were coping, David through activism and Don through seclusion. But days, nonetheless, are (for most of us) numbered."* Don Briggs, Lynch noted, had lived for four years after his initial diagnosis, David Marriage about two. *"But I'm not sure what diagnosis means in either case."*[1]

The 1989 memorial was redesigned to be storable and portable, in the hopes that it could be mounted on other occasions besides Lesbian and Gay Pride Day. But the committee already had its eye on eventually constructing a permanent monument.[2] They hoped to locate it where the temporary memorial was installed, in Cawthra Park, in the heart of Toronto's gay ghetto.

Lynch found the second memorial less aesthetically pleasing than the first. *"Designer John McAuley was something of a lifesaver for us, offering the best design and supervising most of the construction."* But, Lynch said, the final result had *"the colour sense of the paint chips from Canadian Tire."*

Early July found Lynch back at Fire Island, but communal living no longer held the same appeal as it did in the early 1980s. *"Couldn't 'do' the island again without more privacy,"* he told his diary. While there, he got news that his friend Bruce Schentes, in Los Angeles, had developed Kaposi's sarcoma, and that two others he knew had tested positive. Lynch also wrote about seeing an October 1988 *Scientific American* article that had presented a natural history of the disease and made a *"measured prediction that All Will Die."* The article gave him the sense that he was in a very late stage—*"Why go on? The great funnelling clouds the few of us left towards its maw."* Herb Spiers had gone to a Community Research Initiative conference and phoned him on an early July midnight, waking him up to say, "Hang in, Michael, there is good news ahead." Herb reported that clinicians at the conference—front-line people with large AIDS patient loads—were "very encouraged by treatment news and prophylaxis news." The next evening the two of them talked strategies. *"In a time of affliction, who is spared? The patient nearest the good hospital, with an MD willing to move fast and even to anticipate problems and to prophylax. The patient who can get to the leading edge of expertise and work w/it."* Lynch decided that when he was back in Toronto he would ask his doctor, Anne Phillips, an internal medicine specialist, for an appointment, *"to discuss all this."*

Ten days later, back in Toronto, Lynch wrote that Schentes was now in hospital with PCP, and he himself was suffering from chronic fatigue and sleepiness. He cut back on Sinequan, which had a strong sedative effect, and began suffering from insomnia. Lynch, feeling overwhelmed, went to his next AIDS Memorial meeting prepared to quit that group. *"But the tone and pacing of our little group is so pleasant to work with I got interested again,"* he wrote on August 2nd. He cited David Pickard, Alan Miller, Rob Lavery, and Barry Martin as being among the people there who kept him going.

Then, another blow. Lynch was recording events in his diary on August 7, but soon realized: *"I come to the end of the page blocking, I guess, the real news of the day."* Jacques D'Angenais had died the previous night.

> *It is a relief, but one mixed (for me) with guilt: I wanted to visit him more. And mixed w/grief at the way illness crumbled him psychologically, right back into childhood Catholic guilt and family. I didn't know him well even by the time he got sick, but I wasn't ready for the crumble . . . The day I recruited him for the Memorial. His boundless charm, skill and perfectionism in pulling it off successfully . . . Lunch w/him and Gram at Fenton's last Xmas, his crankiness*

and even turning aside from friends. His wheelchair appearance at
Pride Day to see this year's Memorial. A real kid. Another irreplace-
able loss.

Lynch's persistent fatigue was explained just over a week later when
he was, once again, diagnosed with PCP and hospitalized for twelve
days at Women's College Hospital. *"Tuesday night POW! A mounting*
fever." All the ice cubes in the freezer, Aspirins in the bottle, he said,
could not control it: *"crawled into hospital at 7 a.m. and it took 2 days*
to diagnose. Very atypical . . . Stefan, torn, stayed and has been an enor-
mous help." Lynch spent his forty-fifth birthday, August 20, 1989, in
the hospital in a grateful mood. "Thanks to the woman whose labour was
just beginning 45 years ago tonight, to Dot and to PHL III [his father]
and to GPSL [Gail] *who on a Sunday at noon in January 1972 squeezed*
out the person I love more than anyone else ever anywhere, anytime."

He was preparing to teach a course that fall on the American
novelist Willa Cather, and found himself comparing lives: *"My life*
seems promiscuously unfocused, so undirected. I could blame a childhood
that took a long time to overcome, or a setting w/o true support. But Red
Cloud [Nebraska, Cather's hometown] *was Dunn & she made herself*
pretty fast."

The second bout of PCP left Lynch frightened about what was
ahead. He had trouble tolerating AZT, and he wanted *"a working*
antiviral in me before I face the less manageable opportunistics." So he
was determined to secure ddI (dideoxyinosine), an antiviral related
to AZT but indicated for people who had difficulty tolerating that
drug. He would need an underground source. The drug, proven safe
but not yet proven effective, was still undergoing regular clinical trials in the United States. While the Health Protection Branch was
prepared to release ddI under the Emergency Drug Release Program
(EDRP), manufacturer Bristol-Myers was refusing to make it available
until U.S. clinical trials were completed and the U.S. Food and Drug
Administration approved it.

"The struggle for ddI has produced the first confrontation with a
multinational pharmaceutical company," George Smith wrote in the
AIDS Action Now! newsletter. "There is no reason to believe that this
will be the last one, either."[3] The ddI issue opened up a new struggle,

creating a new awareness around problems with pharmaceutical companies, Gary Kinsman recalled. "This was another problem we were up against—it wasn't just the medical profession, the hospitals, and the government." In mid-July AAN! had held a press conference about the lack of access to ddI, and demonstrators set out to occupy the pharmaceutical giant's Toronto offices, located in an office tower at the corner of Bay and Queen streets. By the time the protestors arrived, drug company officials had locked the doors. The protestors blockaded the office, and seven people were charged with trespassing.[4]

Lynch was pretty sure he could get ddI through Herb Spiers in New York, and Dr. Phillips agreed to keep tabs on how he did on the drug, to make sure he didn't get into trouble—if he did get the as-yet-unapproved drug from an underground source. Then Bert Hansen, another New Yorker, reported that epidemiologist friends told him ddI caused irreversible neuropathy. *"Crash! Plummet! So, depression alert. Which means hope alert: I'm drifting into that desperate hope that marks the era Monette describes in Borrowed Time. I need to be cooler."*[5] This entry represents one of the only times in his diary that Lynch mentioned Paul Monette, the author of *Borrowed Time: An AIDS Memoir*, without disparaging him—as, for instance, being interested in people with AIDS "only if they drove Jaguars."

After he was discharged, Lynch began attending the Toronto General's day clinic to be treated with aerosolized pentamidine. Scott Cline was going there as well. *"He's beginning to give up, I think,"* Lynch noted. *"His father's unexpected death, suddenly from a heart attack this summer, has weighed heavily. His miracle deliverer is Compound Q, and he's off to San Francisco to get some when he can. He's been so upbeat—with vitamins and supplements and exercise, for 2 or 3 years. This is a real change."*

Surrounded by so much illness and death, Lynch found the "outside" world becoming increasingly foreign. *"It's gotten hard for me to even imagine that people—on the street, in the ghetto, all over—are leading lives w/o AIDS. Parties, sailing, ordinary worries. They seem unreal."*

With his spirits low, low, low, he decided to ask for a prescription for a "mood elevator." An appointment with Dr. Phillips *"had its usual effect of cheering me up, relieving worry, reducing stress and reassuring me."* Lynch could also take some pride in his role in the community. One Sunday in mid-September he fielded telephone calls from Art Wood (chair of ACT) and Tim McCaskell (chair of AAN!) and got a visit from Bill Berinati (chair of Casey House). *"I felt like an elder statesman, invalid, but flooding with advice."* But, he noted, *"Only Tim asked for such."*

With his friend Gerald Hannon, Lynch discussed plans to scatter Bill Lewis's ashes in David Balfour Park, located in one of Toronto's mid-city ravines and well known among gay men as a site for cruising. *"I realized I couldn't do it. I could never walk back up the hill. He proposes a cab drop and later pickup from Mount Pleasant* [a street adjacent to the low ground of the park]. *Clever Gerald!"* But it wasn't until a year later that the two men managed the task. They ended up on a bridge over the park, *"where indeed we broadcast Bill's ashes. Rather, we poured, the wind broadcast."*

Bodily fatigue was the prime cause of Lynch's depression—at least that's what Toronto psychiatrist Stephen Woo concluded after a consultation in late September. Lynch followed Woo's suggestion that he try taking an amphetamine, Ritalin, instead of an antidepressant.

Lynch wrote to his brother Pat, still living in Dunn, advising him that his planned visit there at the end of the September would probably be his last unless a new treatment significantly improved his energy. "The reason is this. I have precious little energy, and definite priorities as to how I want to use them. They involve doing lectures and readings, establishing the Centre I'm working on here, some travel to visit some friends." He warned Pat to stop expecting visits—that he could only come if his energy levels went up. But he remained optimistic. If he went, he promised, "We'll fish till there's no more to catch—as long as you clean them."[6]

According to Spiers, Lynch's absolute certainty that there was nothing after death led him to place great importance on finishing his work because that, at least, would allow him to live on. "There was nothing else," Spiers speculated years later. "It was total oblivion, blackness, emptiness, the void. He would not entertain any other possibility." Spiers recalled that Lynch said he "found great comfort in knowing that when he was dead, that was all there was."

That month McCaskell's important article, "AIDS Activism: The Development of a New Social Movement," was published in the magazine *Canadian Dimension.*[7] The article highlighted key issues related to the medical system, prescription drug availability, and drug testing—issues thrown into the spotlight as a result of AIDS activism, but which had a much wider significance. McCaskell targeted the lack of any system that would enable doctors to share treatment information and establish treatment protocols. "Over and over one hears that it is patients who are providing information to their doctors in terms of treatment and research. This also means that there is a huge amount of inconsistency in the way that HIV illnesses are treated by different doctors." The article also critiqued the ethics of double-blind placebo trials when they were the only channel for desperate patients to (maybe) get drugs. And McCaskell decried the lack of any follow-up reporting on the effects of drugs released through the Emergency Drug Release Program, and the conflict of interest of clinical investigators, who enrolled patients in trials and counselled them, yet were also being paid by the drug companies that sponsored those same trials.

As George Smith had suggested in his column in *Rites* magazine, AIDS treatment activism was drawing attention to fundamental problems within the health-care system—from issues around clinical trials (who gets to participate) to conflicts of interest and the surveillance of drugs after they were released.[8]

Recruits, "Shit," and the "independent and different power"

During its early years, though AAN! faced death after death among its members, there was also a steady stream of new recruits. When Darien Taylor first made her way to a media subcommittee meeting in the summer of 1989, she was one of the very few women ever to attend an AAN! meeting. After contracting AIDS when she was teaching in Zimbabwe, Taylor had returned to her home in Hamilton thinking that she would, shortly, be dead. In Canada she quickly realized that the thrust of AIDS services was towards prevention, not treatment.

"People were unable to distinguish between prevention and the needs of those of us who were infected," she later said. "My primary

concern was, how do I keep alive?"[9] She first saw copies of AAN! literature at a healing circle that she attended, and she was drawn to the
idea of an activist response to the epidemic. "I hadn't had any political involvement around an organization prior to that. I don't know
exactly what it was that captured my imagination—it might have just
been feeling so completely powerless and alone, that the idea of a
group that was talking about 'power to the people' stuff was what I
needed."

The general absence of women at AAN! was not because there
were no women with HIV/AIDS in Toronto. The AIDS Committee of
Toronto had a women's support group, and Taylor had been a participant. But the atmosphere around AAN! could be intimidating. The
key people in the organization were highly articulate, politically
experienced gay men in their forties, and debate within the organization was often charged and acrimonious.

At the first meeting Taylor went to, Patrick Barnholden was the
chair and Sean Hosein and George Smith were there. "They were
talking and I didn't know what the EDRP was and I remember Ross
Fletcher was sitting next to me and he wrote me a note that said, 'Do
you know what the EDRP is?' and I wrote 'No!'" Fletcher died soon
afterwards, on December 12, 1989, at age thirty-one.

Immediately after the meeting, Smith and Hosein befriended
Taylor and took her to the *Xtra* offices, then located at 464 Yonge
Street, across the hall from ACT, to hammer out an AAN! press release.
Soon she was going to steering committee meetings. In 1990 Taylor
was elected co-chair of AAN! with Glen Brown, in part, she recognized, because "it looked good" to have a woman prominent in the
organization.

While there was definitely fighting and political disagreements
within the organization, there was also a sense of urgency, Taylor
recalled. Relationships with people were often short-lived, not
because people left and moved on, but because they died. "You
worked together, united in your purpose, and maybe some superfi-
cial things melted away in the urgency to get stuff done. Or maybe it
was that we felt that we didn't need to engage in certain things
because we knew we weren't going to be together for a long time."

Among the things that kept Taylor in the work, she said, were the intense and quick connections she made with people, and particularly Pierre Tanguay and Doug Wilson. The relationships "happened really fast, they were really really important and they were over fast." In addition to his work with AAN! Doug Wilson was one of the key people working towards establishing a national PWA association—though in the end the Canadian AIDS Society agreed to have a certain number of PWAS on its board and the push for a national PWA association lost steam. Wilson died in 1992. "There was always a troop of us, you were always going to funerals but you went in bunches and it was like, as one person died, a new person would come into the movement."

Not far away from those thoughts, Lynch was telling his diary in early October: *"I want to write about all sorts of things. But the real power has me write, these days, about facing death, from the deathbed. I'd like to give the world more 'variety,' some laughs, some political challenge, something other than these deathbed meditations. But. And."*

A baseline ultrasound near the end of the month revealed that Lynch had a rare case of PCP—rare because it was showing up not in his lungs but in his bladder. Scott Cline had been diagnosed with the same thing (in his abdomen) about a week earlier. Meanwhile, Gram Campbell had become *"blind as an alley."* In his diary Lynch scribbled out a draft of a long poem, the final version of which, "Shit," was eventually published in a collection on AIDS. In a brief commentary published with the poem, Lynch noted the change in his poetry, the "several sonics not so audible in other of my 'AIDS poems': to indict, to avenge."

> In a system (worldwide, national, local) which simultaneously brutalizes the ill and evades (with far more ingenuity than any lyric) responsibility for brutalization—the buck stops nowhere—one must fix one's target where one can. Injudicious? Perhaps. But remember this: there were well intentioned persons and benevolent rationales at Belsen too.[10]

The poem begins:

The ordinary props of Indian Summer:
lemongrass after the embarrassments of harvest
off-centre pumpkins, maple leaves
like yellow watermelon, vines to prune
while leafless. Unseeing, Gram takes a walk
And David copes with diarrhea. Still sighted,
Scott checks in—our first of extrapulmonary
pneumocyctosis. Gord packs his bags

for home after weeks of no treatment
on the ward, and Ross moves into Gord's room
and Chuck moves over to Casey House.
Musical beds of a sort, but instead of them
growing fewer, we do . . .

Some twelve stanzas later, it finishes:

Wrap yourselves in triplicates, long scarves,
protocols or policy,
we know who you are. Our bodies want
life, our history revenge.
Your patient-management assumed
our patience. No more.

While Security sleeps we take the halls
marking with our shit
the office doors of those
few the angel will pass over.
The rest must go.
Your cleanliness, our corruption.
Your disposable plastics.
Our warm strangling hands.

Lynch had discussed his ideas about mourning and activism with art critic Douglas Crimp, whom he had met a couple of times in New York with Spiers. Lynch had also read Crimp's influential article

"Mourning and Militancy," which explored the discomfort of many AIDS activists with the process of mourning, but stressed the need for *both* activism *and* mourning. Crimp argued that activist antagonism to mourning partly hinged on whether the crisis was seen as "a natural accidental catastrophe—a disease syndrome that has simply struck at this time and in this place—or as a result of gross political negligence or mendacity—an epidemic that was allowed to happen." Public mourning rituals, meanwhile, often seemed to activists to be:

> indulgent, sentimental, defeatist—a perspective only reinforced, as [Larry] Kramer implied, by media constructions of us as hapless victims. "Don't mourn, organize!"—the last words of labor movement martyr Joe Hill—is still a rallying cry, at least in its New Age variant, "Turn your grief to anger," which assumed not so much that mourning can be foregone as that the psychic process can simply be converted.[11]

With AIDS, though, Crimp wondered if mourning had not *become* militancy, since the process of mourning was so often interfered with—as when gay men attended funerals where AIDS or their friend's gayness was never mentioned. "Seldom has a society so savaged people during their hour of loss. . . . Because this violence also desecrates the memories of our dead, we rise in anger to vindicate them."

But not everyone turns their anger into activism. The toll of the epidemic, combined with neglect of the government, had left many affected individuals suffering from numbness or constant depression, paralyzing fear, remorse, and guilt. It is simply wrong-headed for activists to decry those responses, Crimp argued. Gay men must recognize their own terror, guilt, and profound sadness, along with their rage.

In late September federal Health Minister Perrin Beatty announced that ddI would be available in Canada, following a move to make it more widely available in the United States. Bristol-Myers had agreed to release the drug under a new "parallel track" arrangement that gave PWAS early access to promising drugs.[12] At the beginning of November, Lynch began taking ddI. Dr. Phillips had requested it for him under the EDRP, which now promised to release drugs within forty-eight hours. The hospital pharmacy called the doctor's office when the drug arrived, but she was away and it sat in the pharmacy for eight days, while Lynch waited. *"They made no effort to reach the HIV clinic about 20 steps down the hall. Death by bureaucracy!"* he wrote. Lynch finally tracked down the supply himself.

Scott Cline was the next to die. *"I am struck almost as if it were the first. And as dumb as ever,"* Lynch wrote on November 9. *"That sense of an intelligence on a beam w/me, gone. Who'll I talk to about this or that? Scott's efforts were so persistent, informed, non-defeatist."* Just before Cline suddenly reached the final stage of his extrapulmonary PCP, he had received a shipment of Compound Q. Cline was convinced, Lynch noted, that the drug *"would save his life. The poignancy of this near miss."*

Near the end of November, Stefan came home from college at Simon's Rock to visit:

> For me, perhaps for us both, the momentous event was our discussion of what happens if I'm debilitated & need full-time care at home. I've not, in the past, wanted to call on him. But now I do. In the past, he's been pissed that I **wouldn't** call on him, now he knows **I will**. If it takes a year or so out of his education, okay. "A year without education doesn't mean a year without learning," he said. Say it again Michael: Stefan, more than anything else I want to know I can ask you to take care of me when I need care. Now I know that, and am very reassured, happy, peaceful to know it. . . . S wants me to be less "routine" about illness and death, & the surprise to me is that's how **anyone** would read me, especially someone who knows me so well. I interiorize, except for this journal, poems, music. Open up more, M. But his specific request that I rage against the dying of the light—he doesn't (yet) know the poem—still seems one I reject. I'd say to him as I've long said to Dylan Thomas— if father's peaceful, let him be so. If you want rage, **you** rage.

"Fighting Words," an interview with Lynch, appeared in *Xtra* in early December 1989. In it, Lynch argued:

> Narrowing what gay is to AIDS is deleterious. People are dying (not because they're gay but) because the bureaucracy isn't doing its job in terms of providing care. There was certainly death and dying before AIDS, and the gay experience never denied that. The '70s wasn't entirely defined by new discos and parties, so I don't buy

the notion of the party being over. Is there less gay life today? Have people stopped fucking in Balfour Park? Are there fewer clubs?[13]

Lynch also decried the idea of the gay family, because it was based on a heterosexist notion: "I'd like a straight family to see themselves in terms of friends. I'd rather see same-sex friendship be the model to straights. They can learn from us."

During the interview, he realized (and told his diary) *"how gesture after gesture of these 45 years broke with conformity, took (or acknowledged) the independent and different power: but mostly to establish (this was the shock of my mind racing during that interview) new conventions for others."* The Body Politic had become Xtra. The Gay Fathers group, he said, had bored him with its safety—as AAN! had also bored him *"when its presence was secure."* The AIDS Memorial too had become *"far less challenging once we had a public trust in it."*

On January 9, 1990, the eve of Stefan's eighteenth birthday, Lynch taught the first class in his new half-course "Writing the Body." Created and taught only by Lynch, it was "a study of the ways in which a selection of writings since 1860 has represented the human body and developed meanings with reference to it. Literary texts by Whitman, Stein, Joyce, Hemingway and Wittig are supplemented by selected extra literary texts from the medical tradition, popular writing and the usual arts."[14] That week he also heard that Schentes was developing dementia. A few days later, Lynch spoke with Herb Spiers, David Cohen, and Michael Jorgensen about Schentes's deterioration. *"Survivor's guilt may come out of this one for me, but how someone who'd had 2 PCPs can think much about survival . . . How? Simple Hope."*

Lynch's former student and friend George Poland, his wife Ellie Perkins, and young son Ben had gone to spend two years in Mozambique. They were friends of Gram Campbell, knew he was ill, and had sent a letter to him via Lynch. On January 18 Lynch wrote to inform them of Gram's death the day before:

> Yesterday at noon, Alan [Miller, Gram's partner] put a Do Not Interrupt sign on the hospital door and cuddled close for a last chat, assuring Gram that he (Alan) had good support around him and he (Gram) could let go now. When, hours later, he did, Alan

said: "I didn't mean *this* soon!" But it was a relief all round, and a very textbook deathbed in many ways. I'm proud of Alan & the circle of friends that have been around, planning, organizing, and grieving for several weeks now.

Campbell's parents had come from Montreal to Toronto. Their presence, Lynch wrote in the letter, "has been ranging from mildly horrific to vehemently horrific." In the hospital room Lynch had witnessed—or been part of—an "upsetting battle" to care for Gram, which made Lynch stop going in. "Mother fidgeted and father pawed, especially as a way of putting Alan & the rest of us aside. Both parents are suffering, yes, but neither will recognize a shred of common suffering with others." The parents prepared a death notice that would appear the next day in *The Globe and Mail*. When they showed it to Alan, the result was a huge fight. It didn't give Gram's birthday, it made no reference to AIDS, no reference to Alan, and no reference to friends—cancelling out everything his friends knew of him. Alan later showed the death notice to Lynch. "When they leave town," Lynch wrote, "Alan will place another, and Gram will be in it."

Lynch added a postscript to the letter. "A few hours later: A call arrives that my dear Bruce in Los Angeles died of a heart failure about three hours after Gram. A double to the solar plexus."[15]

Amidst all this heartache, there were small pleasures. On January 12, Lynch picked up the first issue of *Centre/Fold*, a publication of the Toronto Centre for Lesbian and Gay Studies—*"After long longing for a product, an image, an announcement of us to the world and (let me repeat) a material something-to-show (for-it-all) product."* Ed Jackson and Lynch had a strong need for that kind of product, Lynch said, fixed *"in the blood, no doubt,"* from their *Body Politic* days. *"This has been an especially long wait."*

There were also felt duties. At the beginning of January Lynch fired off an angry letter to *The Globe and Mail* in reaction to the announcement that the federal government would provide compensation to those who had contracted HIV through blood or blood products.

When it comes to AIDS, Canada's policies remain among the most craven in the world. . . . Now Health and Welfare Minister Perrin Beatty announces that he will compensate some 'victims' to the tune of $120,000 (December 15). Some, but not others. In one stroke he has transformed the craven into the depraved. Even his let-them-all-die predecessor Mr. Epp could not claim such cynicism. . . . The Minister's compensation program oddly accepts responsibility for a "tainted" blood supply even before the development of HIV screening technology, while ignoring its own responsibility to prevent infection in other ways such as education. Some people's health and welfare is a lot more important than others.[16]

Lynch's letter was not published. While his anger was understandable, the compensation issue was complicated and a political landmine.

In the early days of ACT, Lynch had built bridges with hemophiliacs—like the time, at a meeting with Health Minister Keith Norton, when Lynch had turned the floor over to Bill Mindell to argue the need for comprehensive care clinics for hemophiliacs. Mindell later said that in 1989–90 he tried, in his role as a Toronto public health official, to convince Lynch to stay out of the argument about compensation for hemophiliacs: "I said you don't want to be on the wrong side. This is not about favouring one community, it is not about having the disease. This is for malpractice. It is not compensation, it is an out-of-court settlement."

According to James Kreppner, an HIV-positive hemophiliac who would in the 1990s be instrumental in building bridges between the hemophiliac community and gay AIDS activists, the federal government deliberately muddied the water back in 1989. By providing the first compensation package, the government seemed to be implying that hemophiliacs were "the innocent victims" and that it was going to compensate the innocent victims on a compassionate basis. "That really bothered us," Kreppner said, "because that turned people in the general AIDS community against us. And that's not what it was about, and they [the government] knew it. It was about the fact that they were negligent in the way they ran the system—that was quite clear—and in order to forestall legal cases they bought us off."

AAN! was now briefly caught in a turmoil of its own. At the end of 1989 some members had proposed amending the constitution so that those who attended the monthly meetings would set policy for the organization, leaving the steering committee no option but to implement policy. Voting was delayed on the amendment and, in early 1990, it was defeated. The members who voted against the amendment believed that AAN! had to represent the interests of HIV-positive people, and that the organization's procedures, including elections to the steering committee, enabled that approach. "These interests would not necessarily be represented in a policy-setting monthly meeting where the interests of non-HIV positive individuals might predominate," stated a report by Darien Taylor.[17]

The upset prompted McCaskell, in early January, to write and circulate a discussion paper, "AAN! Who We Are." The paper explored the question of AAN!'s relationship to the gay community and to those who were HIV-positive but not gay. The organization had endorsed the importance of maintaining an elected steering committee in charge of policy "as a way of ensuring the dominance of PLWA/HIV people over the organization," he noted. The demographics of the epidemic in Toronto guaranteed a "predominantly gay character" for the organization. Without naming other specific groups known to be affected (for example, hemophiliacs, or IV drug users), McCaskell recommended "affirmative action strategies" to ensure that all people who were HIV-positive or had AIDS were represented in the organization.

Last onsets: classrooms, quarantine, and Queen's Park

The room was packed in late January 1990, when Lynch gave his talk "Last Onsets: Teaching with AIDS" at Trinity College in the University of Toronto. The title hearkened back to the heading —"The last onset"—that he had put on his 1982 diary, marking the period when his mother was dying. "Everyone knew he was sick, and his talk was about what people choose to say when they are near death," recalled David Rayside, a University of Toronto political scientist.

"This business of Famous Last Words makes an interesting study," Lynch argued. But, he added, "As one who has been at more deathbeds during the past eight years than I care to inventory, I'll testify to other scenes. Deathbeds tend to be rather ordinary."[18] Lynch delivered his paper in the funniest way, said Linda Hutcheon, who was in the audience. "He dared us to laugh with him, but it felt very awkward . . . he wanted us to be engaged, but he was not being solemn." Among other things, Lynch talked about his decision to tell his classes that he had AIDS, to "treat the classroom as deathbed." Afterwards, he told his diary: *"No one seemed to recognize the animating force of it: embodied self-reflection, embodied performance."* It was, at the very formal University of Toronto, a high-wire act to promote the idea that "we teach what we are," and Lynch felt some colleagues scowling. *"I felt, by the end, so transgressive in arguing for personal learning."*

A week and a half later, on February 3, Chuck Grochmal, one of AAN!'s founding members, died at Casey House. He was thirty-seven years old. That evening Lynch and some friends went to see *Glory*, a movie about the U.S. Civil War featuring African American partici-pation. *"We were all a mess afterwards . . . How war movies have changed for us since AIDS. 'Us' = those who know it from within . . . the hard part about the epidemic is that no one seems to deal with it. Better put: we, 5 gay men, were agitated by the total and pointless waste of the regiment's splendid body/bodies because of the waste we live through and will be part of."*

That month AAN! staged another protest—this time aimed at comments made by Dr. Richard Schabas, Ontario's chief medical officer of health, about the possibility of quarantine for HIV-positive people. Schabas had recommended to Ontario's minister of health that AIDS be reclassified as a "virulent" disease, a move that would allow public health officials to ask the courts to confine to a hospital carriers who were knowingly exposing others to the virus. Schabas said the measure was meant to deal with extraordinary situations and that it had been endorsed by the Ontario Advisory Committee on AIDS. But in a published newspaper interview Schabas went fur-ther, suggesting that any HIV-positive person having sex, even with a condom and after informing his or her sexual partner, would be vul-nerable to quarantine. "The risk of intercourse with someone who is infected, even when a condom is used, is known to be too high," he said. "My opinion is that the appropriate recommendation or order to someone known to be infected is not to have sexual intercourse."[19]

Schabas's remarks sparked outrage among AIDS organizations, and five hundred demonstrators marched to Queen's Park on February 12 to demand his resignation. The protest attracted a new recruit, Tony Di Pede. An accountant and partner in a real estate firm, Di Pede had never taken part in any demonstrations, and he was still closeted about his sexual orientation. But his lover had recently died of AIDS, and he himself was newly diagnosed. On the day of the protest he was in Scarborough, in the far east of the city, driving to see a client. "I had this big black Ford Sable with leather seats and a car phone, which at the time was a big deal, it was this yuppie thing," he recalled years later. He heard the news about Schabas and the quarantine and the protest on his car radio and was outraged. The protest, he heard, was due to start in a few minutes. "I called my client and said I can't make it, I have a family emergency, I'll explain later, click." He sped downtown to Queen's Park and double-parked—"I said let them tow my car away! I was so enraged about this." At the rally he was the only guy "in a suit and a Burberry's trenchcoat," and he was thinking, "What am I doing here?" He thought people were looking at him like he was an office worker at lunch hour coming to look in on the protest. "I still have the suit, I haven't thrown it out because it was, like, my first protest." He heard Darien Taylor and others speaking—people he would later get to know—and the experience politicized him. Within months Di Pede was treasurer and eventually chair of the board of the Toronto PWA Foundation. The demonstration, too, was a success, helping to stall the decision-making process about whether to reclassify AIDS.

A few days after the demonstration, Lynch went to Durham, North Carolina, to visit Eve Kosofsky Sedgwick. While there, he was casually reading *The New York Times* when he noticed obits for the artist Keith Haring. *"STOP IT—was the heart's cry—LEAVE US SOME DELIGHT IN THE WORLD. And this epitaph ran out my ears: HE MADE THE EYE DANCE . . . Do I especially mourn the talented? Yes, I do."*

Funeral plans and a son's troubles

A section of Lynch's diary—from the month of February 1990—was transcribed and typed out by Rick Bébout and is in the Lynch archives. The excerpt contains Lynch's instructions for his funeral. Bébout inserted some revisions after discussion with Lynch, and there are some handwritten notes from Lynch scribbled on the typed version. *"I do want to control/define the public memorial,"* he wrote. *"No flowers, candles, photos etc . . . As people arrive, no music, only silence. I like such awkward silences, though many resist them."* The second last paragraph of instructions stated:

> We have not mourned enough because we do not know how to mourn enough. From within, the losses are so many and so unstopping and so future, we hardly can deal with it. And from without—even friends or colleagues, oblivious to what's going on next door—no sense of the magnitude and the magnitude—over time.

But Stefan, eighteen, was feeling the magnitude. At the end of March he drove the college van from his campus to Albany, New York, for an ACT UP demonstration, where he briefly saw Herb Spiers. Stefan later told his father that he longed to see Herb—this man he always called his "Aunt Herbeen"—more, and *"to have him, and me around a long time."* Stefan worried that in twenty years there would *"be no one left"* who knew his father, Lynch wrote in his diary. The dean of students, who had been counselling Stefan for depression, snapped at him for taking the college van to a political demonstration. A girlfriend rejected him. Later Stefan took a bus to Boston, *"wandered lost in the financial district, got wet & cold in rain, & eyed doorways where he could sleep. No Y to be found, no hostel. Took the Red Line to Harvard Square, went to see* Lord of the Flies.*"* Later Stefan confided in his father: "Not the movie to see when you're feeling lost and lonely, though I'm not quite Piggy alone among hostile forces." He phoned his dad from the Square, with rain and traffic in the background.

> *"Not an emergency," he said. (It was.) Not so cold & wet. (It was.) Promised to call back in one hour (he did) & I'd arranged for him to stay overnight chez Jack Yeager. He got to Jack's & phoned just now to tell me most of this. I wrote it down to be sure I review all he told me. I wasn't cluing in his first call to the desperation in his laugh . . . Poor kid, wretched and so lonely—it must all be cognate with lack of power to alter HIV, may all be stand-ins for that most powerless fix. Do I worry? Yes. No. I think he'll take care of himself, but I fear that if I were to die tonight he doesn't have adequate resources in himself to deal with his sense of futility, dispossession (of papa & of*

power). I wish he was here, & in a split second tomorrow I would fly to Boston if he needs me, but the day will come when I can't fantasize such protective gestures.

The next morning, Lynch continued in his diary:

I guess it's just sinking in, what S is going through. How I wish I could give him peace and companionship, not just from me but also from others. I wanna make the world safe and comfortable for him. Or do I? Do I want to eliminate his loneliness & loss? Better, give him (what I—we—do give him, as much as any parent can?) the ways to live through the blues. . . . Of course I value them [the blues], especially if they lead to composition . . . I treasure the articulation. The composition. Berryman on Roethke: "Back from wherever, with it said."[20]

Lynch had earlier suggested that his activism and his poetry headed off in rather different directions: the one, a fight for life; the other a meditation on death. But his poetry was now becoming angrier, more political, more explicit. He was working on a long prose poem titled "Alastair Clayton"—referring to the head of the Federal Centre for AIDS and the man whose resignation AAN! had repeatedly sought. In his diary, Lynch drafted a poem that opened with a description from a 1627 anatomy text (Adrianus Spigelius, *De Humani Corporis*) in which a man peeled back his skin the better to see his internal organs. The poem drew comparisons between AIDS demonstrators and victims of famine in Ethiopia, envisioning both as "caricatures of disposability." The limerick-like refrain was blunt:

Alastair Clayton is paid
to make sure we boys don't get laid.

Alastair Clayton takes a just pain
not to cure or to treat, but just to contain

Alastair Clayton offers you tea
from the fruit of the paralysis tree.

Alastair Clayton's silvery hair
keeps him and his boss-man, not us, from despair.

Alastair Clayton maintains his hide
promoting Canadian genocide.[21]

That spring too Lynch was concerned about Doug Bonnell. After the Ontario Conservatives were defeated by the Liberals in 1987, Bonnell had worked as a consultant. From 1989 to 1990 he served as chair of the board of ACT. Lynch had last seen Bonnell in early 1989 in New York at an ACT UP meeting at Spier's loft. Lynch had been in the city to launch his book of poetry, and Bonnell was there to consult Dr. Nathaniel Pier, a well-known AIDS doctor and founder of the Community Research Initiative, which organized clinical trials outside of research centres through the help of community physicians. AAN! had invited Pier to speak in Toronto in September 1988, and the organization commemorated Pier's death—December 27, 1989—in its newsletter of winter 1990.

When Lynch went to visit Bonnell in hospital in Toronto at the end of March 1990 he wasn't prepared for the deterioration he saw. Bonnell had Kaposi's sarcoma, tuberculosis, and MAI (mycobacterium avium intracellulare, a tuberculosis-like condition). He was finding it painful to move his legs but could take a laboured stroll using a tall padded walker. Lynch wrote: *"I will go back mid-week for a real visit. Today I got out fast & burst into tears at the elevator."*

Lynch's diary does not record whether or not he had, as he planned, a longer hospital visit with Bonnell. A week and a half later he was writing: *"Busy days, busy nights. Strenuous times too, with many deaths."* That week he had gone to Bonnell's funeral—attended as well by Conservative MPP Mike Harris and Liberal MPP Elinor Caplan, among others—which had followed *"a sequence including Gram, Jim Bozyk, Chuck St. Chuck . . . I've not let any of them sink in; still haven't 'really' accepted that Bruce is dead."*[22]

ten

TO MAKE DYING GAY

To write history is to write against death. History doesn't stop death—would we really want it to? Would I really want Mammy and Mama still around, to be their child forever?—It doesn't remove its sting, but it does energize the body against simply being stung.
— Michael Lynch, Diary no. 48, May 14, 1985

Michael Lynch taught his last class at the University of Toronto on April 2, 1990. He had decided, after seventeen years at the university, to take a disability leave because of his ailing health. It was a cold, snowy morning and he finished marking essays a half-hour before he had to leave for class. He played the Donna Summer disco hit "Last Dance" (changing the lyrics as he sang along to "last class") and *"danced gamely around the house before going to class, & the dancing let the old stoic floodgates lift a bit. All but weeping when I got to class, and then it was over. Did they know? Some did, in a way."*

Early the next month, Ian Birnie, a man whom Lynch had been seeing on and off for a couple of years, broke up with him. The following night he had a remarkable dream about Bill Lewis:

In the dream I was on a narrow walkway in the airport, and my eye noticed a figurine on sale, and I slipped through the crevice between walkways and fell, but caught myself at the underarms, arms over a rail. On my back, barely holding on, was Bill, holding to me much as I was to the rail. Help came, we were rescued . . . had to convince someone why he didn't have a passport—and then lunched. Michael P., Stefan & 2 or 3 others were along. Bill "looked" very good, healthy, himself, but was very silent. I kept thinking of the stories to tell him (we've almost got the lab named after you,[1] & here you are!), & of explanations that I spent his money and gave away his things, of his dad's death, of choices to defend (you probably won't like the color the front of the house is being painted), of all the odd options now (your apartment is leased, & you can't move in for several months), of anticipating people's reactions (we must warn them or they'll think they're seeing a ghost). Over Swiss Chalet I looked and looked at him, and cried, and was so happy. I hugged him & he let me but was Bill-reticent. Then I thought, what is he experiencing? And asked, but he was mute, and unafraid, but details weren't firm. He'd been a prisoner of war, & was well kept and then flown back to the airport rather suddenly. Others seemed able to cope, or pretend to, w/o turmoil . . . We all walked towards home, Stefan playing catch or something with Bill (Stefan much younger than he is now) & I moved ahead, planning to draw Bill aside for a few considerations before we got to the street. Here, it ended, but rather I left it for a moment, & waking felt like just being in an adjacent room & I could walk back through the door to him . . . sat up, a flood of benevolence and mystery wrapped around me. . . . Now the frets over today's schedule return. I need to cancel everything and deal with this visit. In the dream I wanted to tell him how despite all the changes I think of him daily, and almost daily do the memorializing things. He was benign, even indifferent, but I guess I have guilt? Is this "survivor's guilt"?

In May Stefan graduated from Simon's Rock, and both his parents attended the ceremony. A few days later, the Toronto Centre for Lesbian and Gay Studies held its first awards night, and Ed Jackson announced the creation of the Michael Lynch Grant in Lesbian and Gay History, already capitalized with $8,000 in donations. *"I feel like the monument I've always wanted to feel like—and was truly surprised. . . . Last Sunday I felt so proud of Stefan. Tonight, he said it was his turn to be so proud of me."*

Lynch was in a bad mood when, accompanied by friend Chris Lea, he went away in mid-June to a cottage on Davis Island in Stoney Lake, north of Peterborough, Ontario. *"Michael has been poison,"* he wrote in his diary. *"Driven, obsessed, cranky, unpredictably snappish, ungenerous, obsessive, despairing and despair producing poison . . . had breakdown with Stefan."* Apparently, he told Stefan that he just wanted to quit, to quit trying to live, and then exploded into tears. *"The misery is thinking that you'll remember me as this crank."* Given this mood, Lynch saw himself with a choice: to *"stay in bed or do Ritalin . . .With Ritalin, the management of emotional ups and downs is proving very hard indeed. I say this not to justify but perhaps to excuse."*

At the cottage Lynch penned long, dark limericks and prose poems about death and suicide and families:

> *And did your parents cut you off*
> *on learning you were bent*
> *Why sir, oh no! They love me*
> *They phone me every week*
> *They just don't want me coming home*
> *The neighbours might find out*
> *They sent a cheque to Casey House*
> *a cash donation, rather*
> *You ask too little, girlfriend*
> *more would kill grandmother.*

And his chosen enemy:

> *Like a landscape*
> *engineer*
> *Dr. Clayton's*
> *only mission:*
> *containing the pool*
> *(watch them swimming, thrashing, bleeding)*
> *of infection.*[2]

Back in Toronto, Lynch sat in his garden one morning and wrote: *"Meech lake failed, the HIV confer in SF produced no major hopes for treatments."* The day before he had stayed home from the annual Pride Day to work on the *Lesbian and Gay Studies* newsletter put out by the MLA gay and lesbian caucus. *"The blue geraniums flourish still,* *though the centaurea finally retired. Blue salvia is stately & long blooming: I might get more. Happiness today will be an hour or two to prune and rest, prune and rest. Florabundant, **vine**-abundant, the garden says: come out of your closet-study & love me."*

At the end of June Lynch was bemoaning an agreement to speak at a Toronto meeting of the Canadian Public Health Association. He felt anxious and unprepared for it. The workshop title was "Public Health—Gay and Lesbian Health: Enemies or Allies" and others on the panel were Art Wood and Eilert Frerichs, chaplain at the University of Toronto. Lynch realized, however, that *"things I think **everyone knows** will, in fact, be news."*

The following day he was off on a trip that would culminate in a stay—with Alan Miller, Ed Jackson, and Sam Carvelli—in Willa Cather's cottage on Grand Manan Island, New Brunswick. Lynch took the tiny main-floor bedroom in "Orchardside," the late-nine-teenth-century cottage with its weatherbeaten cedar shingles and *"no noises tonight from anywhere . . . pitch black: no human lights to be seen. Here at last."* He felt he had to *"recoup a little strength and yield a bit to weakness and enjoy the absence of telephones, neighbours, radio, TV and plastics."* While Lynch was there, the landlady brought an older couple to see the cottage. The man looked "like Faulkner" and the woman had a "British way of speaking." The couple, en route to their Cape Breton home, turned out to be Claude Bissell, a former president of the University of Toronto, and his wife. "I teach in your institution," Lynch told him.

Lynch rested up during his Grand Manan stay and, when he had the energy, continued his reading and research into Cather, inter-viewing some of the locals. Meanwhile, Stefan had gone off to Laval University in Quebec, to spend part of the summer taking a French course. On the eve of Stefan's arrival home, in early August, Lynch wrote him a long letter "asking for a full commitment to taking responsibility for me when the time comes." Lynch said he was grap-pling with his terror of Toronto General Hospital—the memories of Bill Lewis's bronchoscopy, of Gram Campbell's Labour Day weekend in 1989. What he wanted, he said, was "an Allan Bérubé"— Bérubé had taken full care of his lover Brian, or at least co-ordinated the care. He and Stefan had a lot to talk about, Lynch decided. *"But I got* to a very deep need/fear/demand. When I can't doublecheck the nurses, who will?"

Lynch had another brief vacation at Davis Island on Stoney Lake in mid-August, this time with Eve Kosofsky Sedgwick. Bernie Morin, who owned the island, was also attentive and at one point gave Lynch a foot massage. *"I would like to train all my friends to do just that foot touch,"* Lynch told his diary. After Kosofsky Sedgwick left, Lynch noted that they had *"a cosy week together."* She was an easygoing and "roomy" friend to be with. Lynch had remarked to her how it always shocked him *"how compact and dense and ranging"* her writing was. *"She didn't mind."*

In early September Lynch had news that Pat Bond had been diagnosed with a bad cancer. She would die just over three months later. She always had a party on Christmas, and she died in the afternoon on December 25, as guests were on their way over. *"So it's over. Life was so hard for her. I hardly believe I've outlived her,"* Lynch wrote in his diary after hearing the news.

After the article "Inside the Ivory Closet" appeared in the fall 1990 issue of *Outlook,* Lynch wrote a long letter to the editors of the San Francisco gay and lesbian magazine. The author, Jeffrey Escoffier, was calling for lesbian and gay studies to remain in dialogue within the communities that gave rise to them, and Lynch scolded him for ignoring activities in Canada. Those activities, Lynch pointed out, included two large lesbian and gay history conferences in Toronto— Wilde '82 in 1982 and Sex and the State in 1985—neither of which had a college or university affiliation. Lynch believed that Escoffier had erased the huge effort to establish the Toronto Centre for Lesbian and Gay Studies, "which is completely community-based, has gender parity on the board and in programming, and is dedicated to the many ethnic and racial communities which make up lesbian and gay Canada."[3]

When he went to the Fourth Annual Lesbian, Bisexual and Gay Studies Conference held at Harvard University in late October, Lynch was gratified to receive attention and recognition and "so much love." He delivered his "Last Onsets" paper again and went home feeling "effervescent" about the weekend in Boston. He had reconnected with *"many good friends from all over"* and was impressed by the fifteen hundred registrants, with a noticeably new generation "coming on strong."

That same month Lynch wrote a three-page synopsis, "AIDS: The First Ten Years," as part of a competition to design a permanent AIDS Memorial. Although its main purpose was to make the case for establishment of the memorial, the document provided not only a cogent statement on the course of the epidemic but also a remarkable, and eloquent, analysis of the role of "silence" in adding to the human destruction—an analysis based on years of painful experience. By 1990, Lynch wrote, thousands of Canadians had been infected with the HIV virus, and despite some advances in treatment there was still only one drug (AZT) licensed in Canada as an antiviral—"and its high toxicity makes it unavailable to many HIV-positive persons." But AIDS had become much more than a new type of epidemic illness along the lines of the influenza or polio seen earlier in the century. It had become "overlaid with social, psychological and political meanings." It had become what medical historian Paula Treichler called an "epidemic of signification," with religious, racist, and homophobic forces organized against it. For years governments and health-care agencies in every country in which AIDS had appeared had chosen to ignore the epidemic, "even as its devastations became daily news."

In the United States, President Reagan made no statements about this major health crisis until *six years* into the epidemic. In Canada, it was not until 1989—*eight years* into the epidemic—that Prime Minister Mulroney spoke the A-word in public. His minister of health Jake Epp said (and did) nothing until forced by political demonstrations to speak out in May 1988.

Silence thus marked the official responses to the epidemic. Silence contributed to it. In health and medical policy, this has meant little financing and planning, and even less research. Educational efforts—in the schools, on the streets, on subway transoms—have met opposition from those who wish to suppress such life-saving information. AIDS is made a matter of shame, guilt, punishments.

Against the horror of this official silence, the AIDS movement arose to fight the epidemic. Those who started this movement in Canada were those who were most hit by the death and destruction: gay men. Beginning in 1983, in Vancouver and Toronto, gay

men organized to break the silence, to provide correct information,
to support the ill and the frightened, and to challenge the inaction
of governments and health-systems.

It was only after a group of persons living with AIDS in Vancouver
had made it a national issue that one antiviral drug came to be available in Canada. Other treatments and services had only come about
after groups within the gay communities across the country started
to provide them. And in 1990 the gay communities—"historically
familiar with being silenced, suppressed, ignored and stigmatized"—
remained in the forefront of the fight against AIDS. "We acknowledge
that other stigmatized groups are painfully affected, and seek coali-
tions from them. But we resist any erasure of the leadership our community provides."

The "official silence" had undoubtedly contributed to the epidemic, and this was most obviously so in the case of safe-sex education. But the silence around AIDS, Lynch wrote, also operated on an
individual level, contributing generously to the increase of suffering
and isolation.

> Most Canadian PLWAS find their illness must be kept secret.
> Information, support systems, and care became far more inaccessi-
> ble. If families or friends or neighbours suspected AIDS, rejections
> or denials escalate pain and stress. Survivors routinely erase the
> cause of death in memorial services or death notices.
>
> For the thousands of HIV positive persons, anti-AIDS practices
> in employment, insurance, immigration law and community res-
> ponses contribute to reinforcing the silencing. When Jack knows
> he'll be fired if his employer finds out he's seropositive, or his
> dentist won't treat him, or a social worker is going to jump into
> tracing his sexual contacts, of course he's going to keep his condi-
> tion secret.
>
> This context of silence has shaped much of the strategy to
> fight AIDS. Community AIDS organizations have insisted on mak-
> ing AIDS speakable and visible. All the statistics have less impact
> than a person saying openly: I am a person living with AIDS.

That same context gave a particular purpose to the idea of an AIDS
memorial.

Naming names matters. The devastations of the epidemic get lost when it becomes a scoresheet, of anonymous body counts of "victims." But the listing of names has an irreplaceable impact in the fight against AIDS—particularly within the communities hardest hit.

Grief too has been isolated by this epidemic. Much as early AIDS organizations sought to establish a community of response to misinformation and inaction around the illness, the Memorial seeks to recognize the communal context of grief, mourning, and remembrance. Even if only a small proportion of the dead may be listed by name, the experience of memorial efforts (for example, the Quilt in the USA and the AIDS Memorial in Toronto) show the tremendous power of naming names as a means of humanizing the massive losses in a way that statistics can never achieve.

An AIDS Memorial performs a number of critical individual and social functions. It gives a focus for personal and public grief. It counters the silencing and denial, the isolation and rejection, that so often mark the experience of PLWAS . . . .

The Memorial, finally, is much more than a quiescent memory. Its identifiable presence contributes directly to the communal awareness that is necessary to lessen the great sufferings ahead for many people. Unlike a war memorial, where there is a definite end after which the structure is built, an AIDS memorial will do its services even in the thick of the epidemic.

Some day it will be possible to list the last death from AIDS. But in the meantime, over the next decades, the suffering of the ill and the surviving will be diminished by the AIDS Memorial. In it, a community of grief takes form. The struggle against the silence and suppression gets a focus. Erected within the turbulent midst of a terrible epidemic, the Memorial thus helps bring it to an earlier end.[4]

Michael and the care team: "we did it well"

In December Stefan was home from college and struggling, alone, to care for his ailing father. His mother was not there to help support him, and Lynch made his son promise not to put him in hospital. Stefan later said that at the time he was proud that his father had made him promise; but later he was angry about having such a demand placed on him.

Lynch was having a hard time:

I've almost given up twice in these last weeks. ALMOST. When there's no energy there's no fight, and no determination. What sustains is touch and affection. True. Amid all these fevers, aches, nauseas, diarrheas, pills, capsules, infusions, shots, i.v.'s, and lassitudes, the greatest threat is panic: agitation, fret. It wears me away like the sea against limestone. The only cure, or at least treatment, is for someone to hold & cuddle me . . . If you want to hold me, hold me.

On Christmas day Allan Miller and Stefan made a stuffed crown roast of lamb, and several good friends came over. Friends promised to stay with him the next day, and on Christmas evening Lynch wrote: "*I am loved. But as* [Victor?] *said on his deathbed: "I know you all love me, but why is no one holding my feet."*

By January Lynch's health had declined enough that his son and his friends set up a formal care team—dubbed the "Lynchmob"—to care for him in his home. "The boys stepped in to help and I was so grateful," Stefan recalled. The team had more than thirty members: a list dated March 31, 1991, had thirty-eight names on it, and most of them were regulars. The helpers included many of Lynch's oldest friends—Rick Bébout, Ed Jackson, Gerald Hannon, Robert Trow, Bill Berinati—as well as his former lover Sam Nirenberg, neighbour Miriam May, and some newer friends such as Helen Reeves, filmmaker John Greyson, and artist Robert Fones and his wife Elke Town. Team members Richard Mehringer, Nirenberg, and Hannon provided regular tactile support, climbing into bed with Lynch, cuddling and sleeping with him. For quite some time Lynch had been unable to climb the stairs to his second-floor bedroom perch, so he had taken over Stefan's old main-floor bedroom, which had sliding doors opening to the back garden.

The team continued their full-service, three-shift-a-day work for six months—an extraordinarily long time for that kind of team care to be sustained. At the beginning no one expected Lynch to live quite that long. And from the first the members of the group kept daily notes recording the coming and goings of the care-team regulars and their observations, Lynch's activities, and the names of visitors. The notes eventually filled two binders.[5]

"To me, the care team was a kind of Cadillac payoff for his work in setting up ACT," Jackson said. "So we pulled out as many stops as we could of people to do it." The team was set up with the help of Yvette Perreault, a counsellor at ACT experienced in such matters, and the members were trained by a nurse, Andrew Johnson, for their roles as caretakers. They met regularly on Sundays.

Absent from the team was Lynch's long-time friend Alan Miller. But Miller, a regular visitor, wrote in the book on February 4: "I have an aversion to crowds so I go in and out as I feel. ML has slapped my hands several times for doing that but I accept the reproach and continue to act as I've always acted." Miller noted that he was reliving the previous year's loss of his lover Gram Campbell, and it was difficult to deal with the present. "There are so many things I just put out of my mind, mostly in defence. Now I see them again and I panic in those memories, and then Michael opens his eyes, smiles, and it's the old Michael. God, it's hard."

In January Bert Hansen visited from New York to discuss Lynch's ideas for completing his book on New York gay history, still tentatively titled "Age of Adhesiveness."[6] George Poland and Ellie Perkins were back from Mozambique for a month or two, awaiting the birth of a second child, and they visited regularly. At the end of January Gail Lynch visited from California. Stefan, who had left college in the United States, announced to her that he was in Toronto "for the duration."

Lynch, suffering from disorientation, decided to go off his medications and prepare to die. A typed note dated February 1, 1991, and taped to the care-team logbook, read: "Michael has decided to stop taking most of his medications and eating food. He wants people to understand that he does not want to go to the hospital again, nor does he want to be resuscitated should he be near the end. *Do not call 911 if Michael dies.*"

After that Lynch was in bed most of the time, with fatigue, chills, incontinence, and night sweats. On February 6, care-team members told him of the death of Michael Smith, who had been an active member of AIDS Action Now! In the middle of all this death, Perkins gave birth to Ned Poland, a younger brother to Ben, whom Lynch had been so taken with. The event was recorded February 9 in the care-team book by Eve Kosofsky Sedgwick, who was visiting from the United States. Bob Reinhard was also in town, from San Francisco.

Despite his plans, Lynch's health had improved slightly by the end of February. His moods in this state, though, were sometimes trying to his care team. In early March he insisted on attending one of the team's meetings and was "unpleasant and rancorous," according to Jackson's note. Afterwards, he was apologetic. According to the care-team notes, he said "he hates himself when he gets that way and will try to avoid it."[7] He told Nirenberg a few days later that he was "tired of not being in control." At a group meeting on March 11, without Lynch, Stefan acknowledged the difficulty that he was having with his father's improvement—"including having to reset my internal date of Michael's death (previously the end of March, now??), wondering if I'll be able, or willing, to return to school in September, etc." Other people, Stefan observed in notes he typed up from the meeting, "shared their issues around Michael's apparent increased lifespan" and therefore their own increased caregiving commitments.

Stefan also affirmed the value of the care-team's logbook: "I see it as part of my inheritance, part of the gay community's inheritance . . . special things that Michael says, or does, or your own thoughts, or whatever, are very important and I value already everything of this nature that is in the logbook." Over the next couple of months Lynch continued to improve somewhat and managed to get out of the house from time to time. But he still suffered from bouts of depression and anger. "Much depression over weakness," noted Hannon on April 3. "Talking about wanting it to end." Lynch had "a sense" that his caretakers didn't "see or acknowledge the extent of his weakness." Ten days later Lynch went out with Bob Wallace to shop for flowers to send to his doctor, Anne Phillips, who made regular home visits. Team member Stephen Atkinson wrote on April 26: "Michael and Robert Trow and I saw and talked a while about problems at the Counselling Centre, and Queer Nation." They also talked about the system at Mount Sinai Hospital's AIDS/Mental Health Clinic. Atkinson noted, "I had the sad thought of what a loss of Michael's clarity, determination and wise leadership it will be."

At the beginning of May Lynch went for two nights to a country inn with Kosofsky Sedgwick and Roger Spalding, a friend from *Body*

Politic days. But when Jackson returned to a regular care-team shift, after having been away for a couple of weeks, he sensed "a deeper well of depression and tiredness, almost beyond words."[8] The same day that Jackson made that observation, Kosofsky Sedgwick presented "White Glasses," her essay about Lynch, at a conference at the Centre for Lesbian and Gay Studies at City University of New York.[9] When Kosofsky Sedgwick had decided, early in 1991, to write the essay for the conference she imagined it would be an obituary for Lynch. After all, he had at that point decided it was time to die, and had stopped taking his medications. Some three months later Lynch was still alive and his health had improved. In the meantime, Kosofsky Sedgwick had been diagnosed with breast cancer. She had a mastectomy on February 28, and around that time care-team members noted Lynch's agitation and worry about her. In the end, "White Glasses" was "an act of homage to a living friend"—and a meditation on friendship, illness, and the meaning of AIDS.

Lynch was well enough on May 11 to adjudicate at the competition for the design of a permanent AIDS Memorial, although the effort left him exhausted. At the end of the month, Nirenberg took him on another out-of-town jaunt to the Ben Miller Inn, a fancy resort near Goderich. "Our trip was wonderful. Get Michael to describe it to you," Nirenberg wrote in the care-team log book. "Weather was perfect. Tuesday night—huge spectacular storm—lightning was amazing! It was all in all a very peaceful fun few days and I hope we do it again at the end of the summer." During this period Jackson said that Lynch would have incredibly intense talks with people who visited him. The visitors would understandably experience difficulty dealing with someone dying, especially dealing with this particular person dying, and Lynch would often end up being the supporter. "He was extraordinary," Jackson said. "He became a kind of caretaker of other people."

On June 6, when someone brought Lynch a copy of the program for the upcoming Pride Day, they "both marvelled at it." It was ten years to the day, plus one, after the first public notice of AIDS as presented by the Centers for Disease Control and reported in mainstream newspapers and the *New York Native*.[10] Lynch's brother Pat came up for a visit in early June, and team member Roger Spalding and others were treated to a real North Carolina barbecue.

Lynch's depression continued, off and on. He told Robert Fones that, when he thought about suffering like his own, "he found the most compatible voice in Beckett's characters, who can find no explanation for suffering but are very articulate in their ignorance."[11] On June 21 Atkinson reported that, according to Stefan, the day was one of Michael's worst so far in his fatigue and state of mind. Lynch again spoke to his son about suicide. "First time in a long time, but as tho' it was the first time *ever*, which I think bothered Stefan a lot," Atkinson noted. "Altho much has changed, it's clearly still *Michael* who is with us."

Several team members noted a dramatic turn for the worse in Lynch's health in June, but remarkably he went out to Pride Day with Rick Bébout on the last day of the month. Bébout wrote:

> He hadn't yet sat up that day until Stefan and I got him dressed, so thin now that his 501s—even over his diapers—slipped down his hips as he was going out to the cab. . . . We did well enough on our own, though after two hours of negotiating through the crowds (and negotiating with Michael, trying to make sure I was wheeling him where he wanted) I was a bit pooped. So was he. But I think he enjoyed it, being in the middle of that crowd, the centre of attention whenever we found anyone who knew him—and many people did. He told me he was in no hurry, that this was likely his last Pride Day and he wanted to soak it up . . . wheeling down Church Street he turned back to tell me we'd just passed two very pretty boys.[12]

Four days later Jackson, who had been away for four weeks, noted that "the change in Michael is very dramatic, even from Monday. Hard to imagine he went out to Pride Day for several hours."[13]

Lynch was lucid and welcoming with Bob Wallace on July 6, but after that he began sleeping a lot. "After taking direction from Michael himself for so long, it's strange to assume that role now," wrote Robert Fones after an evening shift—"a cool, clear night"—on July 8. "His limbs twitch and tend to retract to a fetal position."

Michael Lynch died on July 9, at 2:50 p.m. Stefan and Gail Lynch were with him; Ed Jackson arrived and went into the bedroom just after the moment of death.

"Michael was absolutely the most alive person until the day he died," Gail said. "He was so alive, still talking and chewing on ice and answering questions as he died, and he knew he was dying because he was fully conscious, so he didn't even fade out. He was fully conscious, and then he died." Care-team member Jeff Braff noted in the logbook: "Michael died on my shift . . . Good rest, sweet man. God bless you. The fight will be won because of fighters the likes of you. Your legacy lives on. Be proud of what you have given us. I miss you already."

Friends gathered at the house, among them Bébout, who later wrote:

> The one moment that caught me today was just before I left: Alan Miller leaning over the arm of one of Michael's sleek black leather sofas, looking out the door to the garden. Four years and a month ago we had a birthday party for Gerald in that garden. We were all there then, Alan with Gram, Bill Lewis, Michael, all the rest of us, in Bill and Michael's garden. And here we were in Bill and Michael's house—but no Gram, no Bill, no Michael anymore. Still, we did it well. The team stayed together, Michael was taken care of right to the end, died at home where he wanted to die.[14]

The politics of a community

In his prescient November 1982 article in *The Body Politic*, Lynch wrote of the necessity of making dying gay. Certainly, he himself accomplished that. He was cared for to the end by his whole family— male and female friends, former lovers, and his son and former wife. Lynch had written:

> Gay men drink and trick together, but die alone. We respond to illness by distancing ourselves—by not phoning, by yielding to medical mediators or by frenzied, irreflective fundraising. . . . Once we see this, we may take our lives and our self-definitions back into our own hands. We have to make illness gay, and dying gay and death gay, just as we have made sex and baseball and drinking and eating and dressing gay. This is the challenge to us in 1982.[15]

Stefan said it was the idea of making dying gay that lingered for him. "His death was the epitome of that. So what do we mean by making dying gay?" The son's answer to that question was, of course, informed by his father's thinking. "To him especially gay meant a break from traditional family and a re-emphasis on bonds of affection and not bonds of blood. A sense of brotherhood which goes along with that." It meant forming and building and maintaining a community, establishing connections, achieving "a broader vision for how the world could dig itself out of regionalism and tribalism and into a sense of the fabulous." But more: "When you make something gay, you acknowledge the sexuality in daily life. You acknowledge that there are layers, how you dress, behave, that a broad range of feelings are linked to you and your community's sexualities . . . you absolutely accept your sexuality and that of others around you as integral and important and wonderful." It meant, as well, acknowledging and accepting "the authority of a community of friends and the ability of that community to deal with death," Stefan said. "Acknowledge the dying are sexual, especially since this was a disease linked to sex—don't let this scare us away from our sexuality."

The broader vision of a politics of community took hold in these relatively small but expanding circles in those years from June 1981 to July 1991, and beyond. At a 1988 meeting with AAN! members, for instance, provincial officials had asked why AIDS patients do more complaining about the treatment they receive than, say, cancer patients—which caused George Smith to remark: "This is an interesting question. The more I become immersed in the underworld of AIDS treatments, the more I wonder if everyone who is sick with a life-threatening disease has the same problems that AIDS patients do."[16]

Smith's rumination is apt—and not only because of Lynch's questions of silence and the idea of "epidemic of signification" that Treichler had pinpointed. Many disease groups have since gone on to adopt some of the policies and tactics developed by AIDS activists. But it was AIDS activists who challenged the medical care and research systems and changed them, and there are some good reasons for that. Cancer patients did not suffer from the same degree of stigmatization as those suffering from this mysterious illness that was linked to the twin societal taboos of homosexual sex and illegal injection drugs. "Why didn't you tell us you're a hemophiliac?" a nurse in a downtown Toronto teaching hospital asked activist James Kreppner when he was in hospital with an AIDS-related illness in the 1990s. "We would have treated you much better."

Unlike cancer, AIDS was almost exclusively striking down people in their young adulthood, and in the prime of life. Quickly. Fear and anger fuelled the urgency and vehemence of the activists' demands. Meanwhile, gay men with AIDS were well prepared to do battle. Many were white and middle-class, some with positions of authority and privilege. Many were politically savvy and had fundraising abilities, or at least the confidence to try it. They had political will and resources. Most importantly, they came from a pre-existing community that had been defined through the gay liberation struggles of the 1970s and early 1980s. And, particularly in Toronto, that community had coalesced as a result of attacks from authorities. They could act collectively (unlike, for example, cancer patients). Most of them had gone through the often painful experience of coming out, and in the process they had learned to question authority. Many of them already had an analysis of society's power structures. Finally, they were also both insiders and outsiders, experts and activists. They could meet with and talk the language of bureaucrats and scientists, and they could also rally the troops for large noisy street demonstrations that embarrassed the government into action.

Last words

Michael Lynch, one imagines, would have liked to have the last word in this book. And so we oblige, transcribing the final two entries that he made in the last volume of his sixty-five-volume diary.

22 May 1991. Does anyone know what kind of dreams Shakespeare dreamt while writing King Lear?

23 May 1991. In the dream, I was an architect directing/designing a series of buildings whose basic plans were letters of the alphabet. Starting with a building in the shape of an A, then to B, etc. R was the only hard one, though K was next hardest. Companies and cities heard about the project and made "requests" for certain letters: A was commissioned by Alcan, for example, and K by Kitchener for its city hall. All was iffy at first—it seemed like such a strange and complicated idea, but by the time I woke up it was almost finished and I knew I could die before completely finishing it. Eve was here yesterday and (between sleeps) we talked about projects and (not) finishing them.

NOTES

PLEASE NOTE: Unless otherwise noted, statements attributed to particular people come from interviews or e-mail, phone, or other personal correspondence with those people—as named at the beginning of each chapter's note section.

Similarly, any statements or thoughts attributed to Michael Lynch, unless otherwise noted, come from his diaries, to be found in the Canadian Lesbian and Gay Archives (CLGA), Toronto, accession 96-163/06 to 96-63/11.

one A Political Body

Interviews with Stefan Lynch, Gail Lynch, Paul McGrath, and Robert Wallace. Michael Lynch diaries, no. **17** (Jan. 7, 1981–March 18, 1981), **20** (May 15, 1981–May 27, 1981), **25** (Aug. 20, 1981–Aug. 22, 1981), **27** (Dec. 4, 1981–Feb. 4, 1982), **31** (June 20, 1982–Aug. 12, 1982), **32** (Aug. 20, 1982–Sept. 6, 1982), **33** (Sept. 6, 1982–Oct. 23, 1982), **38** (Aug. 17, 1983–Oct. 15, 1983), **39** (Oct. 15, 1983–Dec. 10, 1983).

1. Michael Lynch, "Living with Kaposi's," *The Body Politic*, November 1982; emphasis added.
2. Spiers always got on well with Stefan—Stefan still calls him his "Aunt Herbeen."
3. The June 5, 1981, item appeared in *Morbidity and Mortality Weekly Report*, published by the Centers for Disease Control, Atlanta. The second item, "Rare Cancer Seen in 41 Homosexuals," *The New York Times*, July 3, 1981, was based on an article in *Morbidity and Mortality Weekly Report*, July 4, 1981 (the *Times* reporter must have seen an advance copy). The subhead for the *Times* article stated: "Outbreak Occurs among Men in New York and California—8 Died Inside 2 Years." See also Mirko Grmek, *History of AIDS: Emergence and Origin of a Modern Pandemic* (Princeton, N.J.: Princeton University Press: 1990).
4. Lawrence Mass, "Cancer in the Gay Community," *New York Native*, July 27, 1981; Larry Kramer, "A Personal Appeal," *New York Native*, Aug. 24–Sept. 6, 1981, cited in Larry Kramer, *Reports from the Holocaust: The Making of an AIDS Activist* (New York: Penguin Books, 1990), p.8.
5. Much of this early information comes from an interview with Gail Lynch.
6. From an interview with Gail Lynch.
7. See Rick Bébout's website, *Promiscuous Affections: A Life in the Bar* <www.rbebout.com>, which provides an inside account of *The Body Politic* and Toronto gay life. The Canadian Lesbian and Gay Archives (CLGA) also has a hard copy on file.
8. Gary Kinsman, *The Regulation of Desire: Homo and Hetero Sexualities*, 2nd ed. (Montreal: Black Rose Books, 1996), p.265.
9. Tom Warner, *Never Going Back: A History of Queer Activism in Canada* (Toronto: University of Toronto Press, 2002).
10. Vanessa Baird, *The No-Nonsense Guide to Sexual Diversity* (Toronto: New Internationalist and Between the Lines, 2001), p.21.
11. Donald W. McLeod, *Lesbian and Gay Liberation in Canada: A Selected Annotated Chronology 1964–1975* (Toronto: ECW Press and Homewood Books, 1996);

Kinsman, *Regulation of Desire*; and also Nancy Nicol, *Stand Together*, a documentary film, 2002, about the gay liberation movement of the 1970s and early 1980s in Canada.

12. Warner, *Never Going Back*, p.136.

13. "Forgotten Fathers" was also published in an anthology: Ed Jackson and Stan Persky, eds., *Flaunting It! A Decade of Gay Journalism from The Body Politic* (Vancouver and Toronto: New Star Books and Pink Triangle Press, 1982).

14. Sheri Zernentsch, "Gay Families in the Media in the Age of HIV and AIDS," M.A. thesis, Communications Studies, Concordia University, Montreal, 1998, p.62.

15. Michael Lynch, "The End of the 'Human Rights' Decade," *The Body Politic*, July 1979.

16. Edward Jackson, in Canada, *Commission of Inquiry on the Blood System in Canada* (Krever Commission), Testimony before the Commission, vol. 109, March 29, 1995. The Testimony, part of the background papers to the Commission, is available from the National Archives, Ottawa, in CD format only.

17. Jackson, in Canada, *Commission of Inquiry on the Blood System*, Testimony.

18. This background comes largely from Rick Bébout, "Trials: A Chronology of the Trials of *The Body Politic*, 1977–1985, with other contemporary events including bath raids, protests and related court cases and the trial of Kevin Orr," Toronto, Dec. 30, 1985.

19. The 1981 bathhouse raids and subsequent protest were covered in the documentary film *Track Two*, Keith, Lemmon, Sutherland Communications Corp., Toronto, 1983.

20. Rick Bébout, "*The Body Politic* and Visions of Community," a paper for the Queer Exchange course on community organizing, November 1995.

21. "'Gay' Cancer and Burning Flesh: The Media Didn't Investigate," *The Body Politic*, September 1981. For an annotated bibliography of AIDS coverage in *The Body Politic*, see Mark L. Robertson, "AIDS Coverage in the Body Politic, 1981 to 1987: An Annotated Bibliography," *The American Review of Canadian Studies* 32,3 (Autumn 2002), pp.415–31.

22. Peter de Vries, "Medical Detectives Lured by Mystery 'Gay' Cancer," *The Medical Post*, Feb. 9, 1982. The article states that at the time the U.S. Centers for Disease Control had records of only one Canadian with Kaposi's sarcoma: a young gay man from Montreal who was diagnosed in New York. According to an April 1982 article in *The Advocate*, Dr. Gordon Jessamine, chief of field epidemiology at the Laboratory Centre for Disease Control in Ottawa, said the Montreal case had not been reported to him. Nathan Fain, "Is Our 'Lifestyle' Hazardous to Our Health? Part II," *The Advocate* 339 (April 1, 1982).

23. Ibid.

24. Pat Sullivan, "The Disease That Transformed Medicine: AIDS Turns 20," *The Canadian Medical Association Journal* 166,6 (March 19, 2002).

25. The issues of *Gays in Health Care Newsletter* cited here are in the serials collection, Canadian Lesbian and Gay Archives (CLGA), Toronto.

26. Diary 32 covered the period from Aug. 20 to Sept. 6, 1982. "The Last Onset" was the title Lynch gave to his completed diary from this period.

27. Peter de Vries, "AIDS Hysteria Seems Unfounded: 'Gay' Syndrome Now Seen in Heterosexuals," *The Medical Post*, Nov. 16, 1982.

28. Nathan Fain, "Coping with a Crisis: AIDS and the Issues It Raises," *The Advocate* 361 (February 1983).

29. Fain, "Is Our 'Lifestyle' Hazardous to Our Health?"

two Blood and Stigma

Interviews with Harvey Hamburg, Robert Wallace, Robert Trow, Stephen Atkinson, Herb Spiers, and Ed Jackson. Michael Lynch diaries, no. **36** (March 2, 1983–May 24, 1983), **37** (May 24, 1983–Aug. 17, 1983), **38** (Aug. 17, 1983–Oct. 15, 1983), **48** (April 20, 1985–July 26, 1985).

1. The Positive Parents flyers are filed under "Positive Parents" in the vertical files collection, CLGA.
2. The figure of 50,000 was the estimate used in 1983 by the City of Toronto Public Health Department. See Joan Hollobon, "Toronto Plots Strategy for Dealing with AIDS," *The Globe and Mail*, July 1, 1983.
3. The Gay Community Appeal—later called the Lesbian and Gay Community Appeal—is a kind of "Gay United Way," supporting causes in Toronto's lesbian and gay community.
4. Michael Lynch papers, accession 91-162/07, CLGA.
5. Michael Lynch, "This Seeing the Sick Endears Them," *The Body Politic*, March 1983.
6. For example, re the Nathan Fain article in *The Advocate*: draft of letter in his Diary no. 35, Feb. 11, 1983; and re Lawrence Mass ("The Case against Medical Panic," *New York Native*): draft of letter in Michael Lynch papers, accession 90-008/09, CLGA.
7. Robert Trow, "Gay Rep to Help Decide Who Will Get Vaccine," *The Body Politic*, December 1982.
8. *The Facts on AIDS*, produced by Barry Spillman, a Gayblevision special, Vancouver, probably late fall 1983, includes footage from the March 12 meeting in Vancouver. Gayblevision videotape, available at the offices of the AIDS Committee of Toronto (ACT). Some of the original organizers in Vancouver were Ron Alexander, Gordon Price, Mike Maynard, Geoff Mains, Noah Stewart, Daryl Nelson, and Bob Tivey. See also the brief description in Randy Shilts, *And the Band Played On: Politics, People and the AIDS Epidemic* (New York: Penguin Books, 1988). For more on AIDS organizing in the Vancouver gay community, see Michael F. Brown, *Replacing Citizenship: AIDS Activism and Radical Democracy* (New York and London: The Guildford Press, 1997).
9. *Gays in Health Care Newsletters*, serials collection, CLGA.
10. *American Association for Human Rights Newsletter*, November–December 1982.
11. For the conference, see Mark Fuerst, "Homosexual Practices Linked to Kaposi's Risk," *The Medical Post*, April 19, 1983.
12. Patricia Hluchy, "Killer Disease Linked to Blood: Evidence Points to Contagious Agent in Mysterious Illness," *The Toronto Star*, Jan. 15, 1983.
13. The relationship between the gay community and the Red Cross would, years later, be well documented in the course of the Commission of Inquiry on the Blood System in Canada. See Canada, *Final Report: Commission of Inquiry on the Blood System in Canada* (Honourable Mr. Justice Horace Krever, Commissioner), 3 vols., Ottawa, 1997.
14. Ed Jackson, "Red Cross: Resisting AIDS Panic," *The Body Politic*, March 1983. In his rush to discredit Newton, Jackson apparently chose not to mention "suggestions" (if not "medical evidence") that AIDS can be spread through blood transfusions and blood products. Four months earlier, in the November 1982 issue of *The Body Politic*, Bill Lewis noted that in July 1982 the Centers for Disease Control reported on three cases of PCP in hemophiliacs. "To prevent bleeding, hemophiliacs require several injections of blood clotting factor per week, and this factor is prepared from the blood of many individual donors. This suggests

that an infectious agent was acquired from the donor's blood." Not hard evidence perhaps, but important enough to raise the issue. Meanwhile, by the beginning of April 1983, AIDS was being declared the second leading cause of death among U.S. hemophiliacs. At the time, eight cases of AIDS had been confirmed among hemophiliacs in that country. See Katherine McRae, "AIDS Big Danger for Hemophiliacs," *The Medical Post*, March 8, 1983.

15. For the Curran quote and the description of the U.S. situation, see Fain, "Coping with a Crisis."

16. Dr. J.B. Derrick, advisor regulatory affairs and good manufacturing processes, to Dr. M.G. Dave, memo, March 8, 1983; UPI, "Red Cross Barring Some for Blood," *The New York Times*, March 7, 1983; and Terry Murray, "AIDS: Come out of Closet, Donors Urged," *The Medical Post*, March 8, 1983. By 1985–86 Murray had convinced *The Medical Post* to let her follow the issue full-time. Her boss, news editor Gary Allen, was a hemophiliac (he died in 1986). Although Allen mostly encouraged her early reporting, Murray said, sometimes he told her to pull back because he was distressed by the news.

17. From the personal papers of Ed Jackson.

18. Jane Gadd, "Fatal Disease Feared, High-Risk Groups Asked Not to Donate Blood," *The Globe and Mail*, March 10, 1983, bulldog edition; and Jane Gadd, "Fatal Disease Feared, Groups at Risk Advised Not to Donate Blood," March 10, 1983, subsequent editions. See also Canada, *Commission of Inquiry on the Blood System*, Testimony, vol. 109.

19. A.V. Miller, *Gays and Acquired Immune Deficiency Syndrome (AIDS): A Bibliography*, publication no.7 (Toronto, Canadian Gay Archives, 1982). Miller produced this bibliography while working in the Ontario Ministry of Labour Library. He had produced previous bibliographies on homosexuality and employment for that library, which was trying to build up its collection on human rights and occupational health and safety. "Most of the gay press [which was early off the mark covering the epidemic] wasn't indexed, so the bibliography helped index the large gay press that the public didn't know existed." Requests for the bibliography came in from around the world. Following the first edition, there was a 1983 edition and an expanded 1985 edition, "which dropped most of the medical sources since by then medical indexes were very good." Personal e-mail from Alan Miller, Nov. 16, 2000.

20. Document in Bill Lewis papers, accession 87-019/06, CLGA.

21. The Canadian Hemophilia Society (CHS) is not aware of any Canadian hemophiliacs being infected with HIV through blood or blood products after 1987.

22. A copy of the release is item no.38 in Gay Community Documents, an exhibit prepared by the Canadian Red Cross Society and submitted to the *Commission of Inquiry on the Blood System in Canada*.

23. Terry Murray, "Haitians Charge Racism against Red Cross," *The Medical Post*, April 19, 1983.

24. Correspondence with Dr. Richard Fralick, then associate medical officer of health for the City of Toronto.

25. The list of fifty-two interested persons, collected from the Ryerson meeting, is in the personal archives of Bert Hansen.

26. The actual wording in the final pamphlet, which was distributed at the April 5, 1983, forum on AIDS at Ryerson Polytechnic, can be found in Canada, *Final Report*, vol. 1, p.254.

27. AIDS Committee of Toronto papers, accession 91-112/01, CLGA.

28. "Medical Caution and Political Judgment," editorial, *The Body Politic*, May 1983. Jackson, who wrote the editorial, would later say it was one of the pieces he was most proud of.

29. Tim McCaskell, "Thousands Demand AIDS Funding," *The Body Politic*, July/August 1983.

30. Robert Reinhard, letter, Michael Lynch papers, accession 97-162/07, CLGA.

31. Ed Jackson, "Fed's AIDS Task Force Excludes Risk Groups," *The Body Politic*, June 1983. The announcement of the task force came on May 5, 1983. It would be another three months before a National Advisory Committee on AIDS (NAC/AIDS) was announced. It was chaired by Dr. Norbert Gilmore, a Montreal immunologist.

32. Ed Jackson, "Nationwide AIDS Report: Checking up on the Experts," *The Body Politic*, July/August 1983.

33. Arthur Felson and Michael Shernoff, "AIDS Groups Find Solidarity in Denver," *New York Native*, July 4–17, 1983.

34. By 1987 there would be twenty-one reported cases of AIDS in Nova Scotia. As of June 2002, there were 577 reports of positive HIV tests and 295 reported AIDS cases in Nova Scotia and Prince Edward Island, according to Health Canada.

35. Bob Frederickson, in Canada, *Commission of Inquiry on the Blood System*, Testimony, vol. 62, July 29, 1994.

36. The report of the Commission of Inquiry on the Blood System includes a brief rundown of early gay community organizing. While the focus is on disseminating warnings about blood donations, the outline provides a snapshot of activity nationwide. See Canada, *Final Report*, vol. 1, pp.252–57.

37. AIDS Committee of Toronto papers, accession 91-112/01, CLGA.

38. Stephen Fontaine, who died in 1995, wrote an early informative magazine article on AIDS for doctors: Fontaine, "AIDS: Bringing the Gay Patient out of the Closet," *Canadian Doctor*, July 1983.

three Against Hysteria

Interviews with Stephen Atkinson, Bill Mindell, and Bert Hansen. Michael Lynch diaries, no. **37** (May 24, 1983–Aug. 17, 1983), **38** (Aug. 17, 1983–Oct. 15, 1983), **40** (Dec. 11, 1983–Jan. 29, 1984).

1. Significantly, a copy of part of Hamburg's Pride Day address was among Lynch's papers in the Canadian Lesbian and Gay Archives.

2. From Hamburg's speech to Pride Day, in Michael Lynch papers, accession 89-008/01, CLGA, p.3.

3. Lionel Morton, "A Short History of ACT's Brochures," July 31, 1984, in Ontario Gay Community Documents, vol. 139, Part II, 00251-253.

4. Michael Lynch, "Until We Know: Choices Facing the Gay Community of Toronto," speech, Jarvis Collegiate, Toronto, June 29, 1983, Michael Lynch papers, accession 91-045, CLGA.

5. Ed Jackson, "Not a Victim: A 'Person with AIDS,'" *The Body Politic*, October 1983.

6. Joan Hollobon, "Toronto Plots Strategy for Dealing with AIDS," *The Globe and Mail*, July 1, 1983.

7. Hollobon, "Toronto Plots Strategy"; and Ed Jackson, "Grassroots Action; Governmental Vagueness," *The Body Politic*, September 1983.

8. "Disease Victims Relate Stark Tale," *The Globe and Mail*, July 1, 1983.

9. Terry Murray, "AIDS an Emerging Epidemic, Says Toronto Health Group," *The Medical Post*, Aug. 9, 1983.

10. "Stevens" refers to the poet Wallace Stevens. "Ananke" is a Greek term that means necessity, or an imperative, and was used by Herodotus to refer to the forces of history.

11. Jackson, in Canada, *Commission of Inquiry on the Blood System*, Testimony, vol.110.
12. Nick Sheehan, "Toronto Group to Help with AIDS," *NOW*, July 21–27, 1983.
13. Canada, *Commission of Inquiry on the Blood System*, National Hearings, March 1995, Ontario Gay Community Documents, August to December 1983, Exhibits, vol. 139, Part II, p.00062.
14. Tim Lukasewich, "AIDS Hazard in Gays' Blood," *The Toronto Sun*, July 20, 1983; Sheehan, "Toronto Group to Help with AIDS."
15. Derrick to Dr. A. Perrault, memo, Jan. 11, 1984, in Canada, *Commission of Inquiry on the Blood System*, Ontario Gay Community Documents, 1984, Exhibits, vol. 140, p.00027.
16. Dale McCarthy, in Canada, *Commission of Inquiry on the Blood System*, Testimony, vol. 110.
17. Bill Mindell, in Canada, *Commission of Inquiry on the Blood System*, Testimony, vol. 110.
18. Bill Lewis papers, accession 87-019/06, CLGA.
19. The house renovation was written up in *Toronto Life* magazine: Felicite Kirby, "Divide Conquer: How Two People Made Two Homes out of One House," *Toronto Life*, April 1985.
20. AIDS Committee of Toronto executive meeting, minutes, Sept. 27, 1983, in Canada, *Commission of Inquiry on the Blood System*, Ontario Gay Community Documents, August to December 1983, Exhibits, vol. 139, Part II.
21. Canada, *Commission of Inquiry on the Blood System*, Ontario Gay Community Documents, August to December 1983, Exhibits, vol. 139, Part II.
22. Ibid., p.00041.
23. AIDS Committee of Toronto executive meeting, minutes, Sept. 27, 1983, p.00098.
24. Bert Hansen, address to Toronto Public Health Department, Toronto, Oct. 13, 1983.
25. Several documents describing this meeting are in Canada, *Commission of Inquiry on the Blood System*, Ontario Gay Community Documents, August to December 1983, Exhibits, vol. 139, Part II.
26. Rick Bébout, "Is There Safe Sex? Looking behind Advice on AIDS," *The Body Politic*, December 1983.
27. As recorded by Michael Lynch, Diary no. 40, Dec. 20, 1983.

four Swansong to Activism?

Interviews with Herb Spiers and Bill Mindell. Michael Lynch diaries, no. **40** (Dec. 11, 1983–Jan. 29, 1984), **41** (Jan. 29, 1984–March 24, 1984), **42** (March 25, 1984–May 28, 1984), **43** (May 28, 1984–Aug. 8, 1984), **44** (Aug. 10, 1984–Sept. 28, 1984), **45** (Sept. 28, 1984–Dec. 15, 1984), **46** (Dec. 15, 1984–Feb. 8, 1984).

1. Quoted in Terry Murray, "First AIDS Victim to Speak out Now Dead," *The Medical Post*, Jan. 24, 1984.
2. ACT to Graham Ritchie, senior producer of CBC-TV national news, March 19, 1984, in Canada, *Commission of Inquiry on the Blood System*, Ontario Gay Community Documents, 1984, Exhibits, vol. 140.
3. Terry Murray, "Norton Does AIDS Homework," *The Medical Post*, Sept. 20, 1983.
4. Michael Lynch, chair of ACT, to Minister of Health Keith Norton, April 3, 1984, in Canada, *Commission of Inquiry on the Blood System*, Ontario Gay Community Documents, 1984, Exhibits, vol. 140.

5. It is unclear if this press release was ever issued. There is no evidence of a story appearing about it in the Toronto print media.
6. Canadian Hemophilia Society papers, accession 95-115, CLGA.
7. Terry Murray, "AIDS Victor Is a Victim of Politics," *The Medical Post*, May 15, 1984.
8. Steven Epstein, *Impure Science: AIDS, Activism, and the Politics of Knowledge* (Berkeley: University of California Press, 1996), p.71.
9. In 1994 Stefan and Ed Jackson rented a motorboat to scatter Michael Lynch's ashes on the river (see the Foreword here). Lynch's friend Robin Hardy writes about a walk he and Lynch took to the bridge, and how Lynch recounted the history of the bridge, including "how they had invented the technology for the world's first suspension bridge as it was built." Robin Hardy with David Groff, *The Crisis of Desire: AIDS and the Fate of Gay Brotherhood* (Boston and New York: Houghton Mifflin Company, 1999), p.137.
10. "Statement by Michael Lynch, chair, AIDS Committee of Toronto, 4 June 1984," in Bill Lewis papers, accession 87-019/06, CLGA.
11. M.L.A., "Women Talk about AIDS," *Rites*, July/August 1984.
12. Simon Watney, "Safer Sex as Community Practice," in *AIDS: Individual, Cultural and Policy Dimensions*, ed. Peter Aggleton, Peter Davies and Graham Hart (Philadelphia: Falmer Press, 1990).
13. The photographs were published the following spring, in Kirby, "Divide Conquer."
14. Joan Hollobon, "AIDS on Rise: 51 Cases in 4 Months, Ottawa Says," *The Globe and Mail*, Nov. 26, 1984.

five These Waves of Dying Friends

Interview with Sam Nirenberg. Michael Lynch diaries, no. **46** (Dec. 15, 1984–Feb. 8, 1985), **47** (Feb. 10, 1985–April 19, 1985), **48** (April 20, 1985–July 26, 1985), **49** (July 27, 1985–Nov. 25, 1985), **50** (Nov. 25, 1985–March 14, 1986), **51** (March 14, 1986–July 29, 1986), **52** (July 27, 1986–Nov. 12, 1986), **53** (Nov. 13, 1986–Jan. 29, 1987), **54** (Feb. 12, 1987–April 19, 1987), **55** (April 19, 1987–Sept. 23, 1987).

1. Michael Lynch, Diary no. 52, Aug. 7, 1986. I found no evidence, among his papers at the CLGA, that Lynch had actually acted on this idea, and attached the stars to folders, etc.
2. Michael Lynch, "TBP's Hannon and Jackson in *Toronto Life*," *The Body Politic*, June 1979.
3. Quoted in Lynch, Diary no. 48, May 9, 1985.
4. Lynch, Diary no. 49, Nov. 2, 1985.
5. Michael Lynch, "Saying It," *The Body Politic*, January 1986.
6. Ibid.
7. The document was submitted as background to the Commission of Inquiry on the Blood System; see Canada, *Commission of Inquiry on the Blood System*, Exhibits, vol. 141, Part I, document, Ontario Gay Community Documents, June to August 1985; emphasis added.
8. Ibid.; emphasis added.
9. Ken Popert, "AIDS Groups to Hold First National Meeting," *The Body Politic*, May 1985. Other points in this paragraph are from Warner, *Never Going Back*, pp.148–251; Canada, *Commission of Inquiry on the Blood System*, vol. 1, p.255; Ed Jackson, "Facing a Common Enemy," *The Body Politic*, July 1985; and David Henderson, "Halifax: Getting Together to Battle AIDS," *The Body Politic*, December 1984.

10. Picasso's painting is *Blue Guitar*; Wallace Stevens's poem is "The Man with the Blue Guitar."

11. The attitude and behaviour of Ward's parents are criticized in one of Lynch's published poems, "Shit," in *A Leap in the Dark: AIDS, Art and Contemporary Culture*, ed. Allan Klusacek and Ken Morrison (Montreal: Véhicule Press and Artextes Editions, 1992).

12. In the Michael Lynch papers, accession 91-045, CLGA.

13. Rick Bébout, memo, Toronto, January 1986. *Xtra* was originally launched as a supplement to *The Body Politic* in 1984.

14. At the time there was some debate about whether HIV antibodies might remain static and result in symptoms such as night sweats and fatigue, but not progress towards "full-blown" AIDS and the opportunistic infections that were killing people. This was probably what Lynch meant by "subclinical HIV."

15. Michael Lynch, "Putting Rhetoric Aside," *The Body Politic*, June 1986.

16. Dennis Altman to Michael Lynch, undated, Michael Lynch papers, accession 91-162/09, CLGA.

17. After Lynch's death in 1991, the poem was inscribed on the permanent AIDS Memorial in Toronto. "Cry" was also published in *The New Republic*.

18. TAG is an acronym for Toronto Area Gays, an organization founded by Harvey Hamburg in 1975, which ran support groups and a phone-counselling line.

19. Diary, in Bill Lewis papers, accession 91-162/05, CLGA.

20. Lynch's Diary no. 52, for Sept. 30, 1986, records that Bernd called "w/news that my porn pix have been published, but he barely recalled where & hadn't bought one." It has been reported that these pictures were in *Honcho* magazine, but that appears to be incorrect.

21. Ed Jackson, "AIDS: Double Exposure, Ontario and British Columbia Ignore Fears about Confidentiality of AIDS Antibody Test Results," *The Body Politic*, December 1985. *The Body Politic* had extensive coverage of the new test, starting with several articles in the December 1985 issue.

22. Michael Lynch to Gail Lynch, Nov. 6, 1986, in Michael Lynch papers, accession 91-162/09, CLGA.

23. Eve Kosofsky Sedgwick, *Tendencies* (Durham, N.C.: Duke University Press, 1993). "White Glasses" is the title of her essay about Lynch in this volume.

24. Rick Bébout, "What Happened?" *The Body Politic*, February 1987.

25. Spiers's comment on this exchange with Stefan (related to him during an interview) was noteworthy. "[Michael] didn't say 'I don't love you.' He said, 'why wouldn't I want to continue living with my work?'—and that is not a bad legacy for a father to leave his son."

26. "A Week in Nova Scotia" was printed and bound by Rick Bébout.

27. From "AIDS and the Arts," a documentary made for the CBC-Radio program *State of the Arts*, produced by Katherine Ashenburg. The documentary first aired on April 12, 1987.

28. The poem was published under the title "Conspirators" in *These Waves of Dying Friends: Poems by Michael Lynch* (New York: Contact II Publications, 1989).

29. From "AIDS and the Arts," a 1987 documentary for *The Journal* (CBC television).

six The Yellow Glove

Interviews with Ed Jackson, Herb Spiers, and Tim McCaskell. Michael Lynch diaries, no. **55** (April 19, 1987–Sept. 23, 1987), **56** (Sept. 23, 1987–Dec. 5, 1987), **57** (Dec. 6, 1987–March 10, 1988).

1. Judith Knelman, "War on AIDS Intensifies on Several Fronts at U of T," *The University of Toronto Bulletin*, June 29, 1987.

2. The 1984–85 study led to several research papers. The first appears to be Randall Coates et al., "A Prospective Study of Male Sexual Contacts of Men with AIDS-Related Conditions (ARC) or AIDS: HTLV-II Antibody, Clinical, and Immune Function Status at Induction," *Canadian Journal of Public Health* 77 (Supplement 1, May/June 1986). Data from the studies was used in at least two other reports for *American Journal of Epidemiology*.

3. I found no mention in Lynch's diaries that Lewis had told him about having had a test for HIV, or about testing positive. However, one friend of Lewis said that the scientist had frozen his own blood samples for many years and had gone back and tested them for HIV, so that he not only knew he was positive, but also had some idea of when he contracted the virus.

4. Letter to Bill Lewis from his father, July 5, 1987, Bill Lewis papers, accession 91-162/05, CLGA.

5. Michael Lynch, "Here Is Adhesiveness: From Friendship to Homosexuality," *Victorian Studies* 29, 1 (Autumn 1985).

6. Bill Lewis papers, accession 91-162/05, CLGA.

7. The treatment was described in an article in the British medical journal *The Lancet* and the advance in Judith Knelman, "AIDS: No Cure, but Some Headway," *University of Toronto Alumni Magazine*, Autumn 1987.

8. Media release, University of Toronto, Sept. 21, 1987.

9. Lynch later published this poem as a foreword to his own book of poetry, *These Waves of Dying Friends*, which was dedicated to Lewis. Robert Wallace provided me with a copy of an audiotape recording of the memorial service.

10. Hardy with Groff, *Crisis of Desire*, p.164.

11. Canadian figures from Health Canada, *HIV and AIDS in Canada Surveillance Report*, Health Protection Branch, Laboratory Centre for Disease Control, Ottawa, Dec. 31, 1987. Table 17 reported the number of AIDS deaths before 1988 as totalling 1,152.

12. The quote is from a note to "Yellow Kitchen Gloves" in *These Waves of Dying Friends*.

13. Lynch, "These Waves of Dying Friends."

14. Randy Shaw, *The Activists' Handbook: A Primer for the 1990s and Beyond* (Berkeley: University of California Press, 1966), p.215.

15. John St. James, *AIDS Treatment News* 23 (Jan. 16, 1987).

16. Epstein, *Impure Science*, p.218.

17. This state of affairs in documented in a series of letters from Dr. Michael Hulton to federal officials, and a reply to him from Minister of Health Jake Epp. Also, on Dec. 7, 1987, Hulton wrote to Michael Davis, director of clinical trials for the Federal Centre for AIDS, for approval to use aerosolized pentamidine to conduct, with colleagues, a comparative trial of agents used to prevent PCP. His request was refused in a December 24, 1987, letter of reply.

18. Lillian Newbery, "Ottawa Asks 2 Firms to Test Drug on AIDS Symptom," *The Toronto Star*, Jan. 12, 1988.

19. To reach a wider audience, Lynch rewrote his *Xtra* article, and the result was published as an opinion piece in *The Globe and Mail*: Michael Lynch, "Ottawa Fiddles While AIDS Patients Yearn for Help," *The Globe and Mail*, Dec. 30, 1987.

20. Peter Wood to Michael Lynch, December 1987, Michael Lynch papers, accession 91-162/10, CLGA.

21. Michael Lynch to "Sarah," undated but from early March 1988, Michael Lynch papers, accession 91-162/09, CLGA.

22. Chuck Grochmal, "Is Nothing Sacred? TO's AIDS Committee Takes a Lot of Heat," *Xtra*, July 1, 1988.

23. From notes, Greg Pavelich papers, accession 97-029/01, CLGA.

24. The 1,600 figure is from Michael Hulton to Michael Davis, director of clinical trials for the Federal Centre for AIDS, letter, Dec. 7, 1987.

25. Tim McCaskell, "AAN! Who We Are Discussion Paper," Jan. 12, 1990, in Greg Pavelich papers, accession 97-029/01, CLGA.

26. Michael Lynch, "Killing Us Softly: Are Some City Politicians against Safe Sex Education Because They Want Gay Men to Die?" *Xtra*, Nov. 27, 1987. It was around this time that John Greyson's five-minute video *The ADS Epidemic* (1987) appeared, produced as a kind of music-video counter-advertisement (promoted as a "safe-sex video") and satirizing the social response to homosexuality and AIDS. "ADS" stood for "Acquired Dread of Sex."

27. Michael Lynch, "Saying It," *The Body Politic*, January 1986.

seven From Elegy to Action

Interviews with Robert Wallace, Tim McCaskell, Gary Kinsman, Dr. Norbert Gilmore, Dr. Brian Willoughby (Kevin Brown's family doctor), Ed Jackson, Rick Bébout, Dr. Michael Hulton, Sarah Yates-Howarth, and Douglas Elliott. Michael Lynch diaries, no. **57** (Dec. 6, 1987–March 10, 1988), **58** (March 11, 1988–July 3, 1988).

1. George Smith to AAN! members, April 7, 1989, Michael Lynch papers, accession 91-162/10), CLGA.

2. Health Canada, Laboratory Centre for Disease Control, AIDS updates.

3. The quotations from Brown are from a 1986 television interview with Brown by Laurier LaPierre, CKVC TV (B.C.), video copy at the Pacific AIDS Resource Centre Library in Vancouver. For Hilary Wass, see Rob Joyce, "Still in the Waiting Room," *The Body Politic*, June 1986, and Rob Joyce, "Names for Hope," *Angles* (Vancouver), June 1986. See also Rob Joyce, "Life and Love after AIDS," *The Body Politic*, May 1986.

4. From B.C. PWA Society, panel discussion, September 1986, videotape, Pacific AIDS Resource Centre Library, Vancouver.

5. Caitlin Kelly, "Nothing to Lose, Victim Says AIDS Group to Press Epp on Experimental Drug Use," *The Globe and Mail*, June 27, 1986.

6. Lillian Newbery, "Transplant Drug No Help to AIDS Victims, Study Says," *The Toronto Star*, Sept. 25, 1986; and A. Phillips et al. (including R. Coates), "Cyclosporine-Induced Deterioration in Patients with AIDS," *Canadian Medical Association Journal* 140,12 (June 15, 1989), pp.1456–60.

7. Ken Popert, "Feds to Rush AIDS Drugs: Quick Action Promised but PWAS Say They've Heard It All Before," *The Body Politic*, August 1986.

8. Rob Joyce, "Still in the Waiting Room," *The Body Politic*, June 1986.

9. Issues of *AIDS Treatment News* are available on the Internet: <www.Aids.org/immunet/atn.nsf>.

10. At first, in early October, it was announced that AZT would be available only to one hundred patients who participated in studies in Toronto, Vancouver, and Montreal; Lillian Newbery, "Metro AIDS Victims to Help Test New Drugs, *The Toronto Star*, Oct. 2, 1986. Then federal Health Minister Jake Epp announced that the drug would be available to all PWAS who had suffered a bout of PCP—or about 180 people; Canadian Press, "New AIDS Treatment Could Help 180 Patients," *The Toronto Star*, Nov. 5, 1986.

11. Tom Barrett, "AIDS Comment No Slur, Dueck Says," *The Vancouver Sun*, June 11, 1987.

12. For the statements made at the January 28, 1988, press conference, see Bernard Courte papers, accession 91-176/02, CLGA.

13. Letter to Lynch, Jan. 4, 1988, Michael Lynch papers, accession 91-162/09, CLGA.

14. For Fauci's testimony before the congressional committee, see Bruce Nussbaum, *Good Intentions: How Big Business and the Medical Establishment Are Corrupting the Fight against AIDS* (New York: Atlantic Press Monthly, 1990), pp.266–74; and Shilts, *And the Band Played On*, p.616.

15. Ken Popert, "Turning up the Heat: Official Indifference to AIDS Attacked," *Xtra*, Feb. 12, 1988.

16. Interview with Michael Hulton in John Greyson (writer, director, producer), *The Pink Pimpernel*, film, Trinity Square Video, Toronto, 1989.

17. The Dewar quote is from notes taken at the Jarvis meeting by AAN! member Bernard Courte, in Courte papers, accession 91-176/02, CLGA. The subsequent quotes, unless otherwise noted, are from these notes or from Popert, "Turning up the Heat." The Hulton information is from my interview with Hulton. There was also a newspaper feature written about this: Suzanne Morrison, "AIDS on Drug Trial: Sometimes It's Necessary to Break the Law," *The Hamilton Spectator*, April 23, 1988.

18. Ann Silversides, "Face It: Nice Girls Do Get AIDS," *Elm Street* (Toronto), Summer 1998.

19. Michael Lynch to the Editor, *Toronto Life*, June 12, 1990, in Michael Lynch papers, accession 91-162/11, CLGA.

20. Larry Kramer, *Reports from the Holocaust: The Making of an AIDS Activist* (New York: Penguin Books, 1990), p.100.

21. Michael Lynch, "Moving On: Chair Joan Anderson Steps down at ACT," *Xtra*, Feb. 12, 1988.

22. Jackson, Bébout, and Orr produced most of ACT's educational material from 1985 to 1989.

23. Douglas Crimp, "Mourning and Militancy," *October* 51 (Winter 1989).

24. Dr. Herbert Spiers, "The President's Commission on AIDS, Testimony," Feb. 19, 1988, in Michael Lynch papers, accession 89-008/01, CLGA.

25. Coates died Sept. 26, 1991, at age forty-two. He had just recently been promoted to chair of the Department of Preventive Medicine and Biostatistics, University of Toronto.

26. David MacLean, "The Battle against AIDS," *Metropolis* 1,40 (Feb. 23, 1989).

27. Nussbaum, *Good Intentions*, p.233.

28. McCaskell interview in Greyson, *Pink Pimpernel*.

29. "IDEAS about AIDS: A Decade of Reporting about the Science and Politics of an Epidemic, 1987 to 1996," CBC-Radio *Ideas*, 1996, program 5, transcript, p.4. The Dewar quote is from David Adkin, "'Four Will Die': Activists Protest Experiment on PWAS," *Xtra*, March 18, 1988.

30. Greyson, *Pink Pimpernel*. Greyson used footage from the demonstration in his film, a campy rendition of the early days of AAN! intended in part as a recruitment film for the organization.

31. AAN! Public Action Committee minutes, March 29, 1988, in Greg Pavelich papers, accession 97-029/01, CLGA.

32. Allan Bérubé, "Caught in the Storm: AIDS and the Meaning of Natural Disaster," *Outlook*, Fall 1988.

33. Michael Lynch, "The Power of Names: Finding Ways to Remember Our Friends," *Xtra*, Feb. 26, 1988.

34. The reference is to his forthcoming book of poetry, *These Waves of Dying Friends*.

35. "A Tale of Major Betrayal" *AIDS Action News!* 1 (March 1988), in lesbian and gay serials collection, CLGA.

36. From documents and agreed statement of facts in *Brown v. British Columbia* (Minister of Health) (1990) 42 B.C.L.R. (2d) 294 (S.C.); Epstein, *Impure Science*, p.199.

37. Kelly Toughill, "Ottawa Blocks Sale of Untested Anti-AIDS Drug," *The Toronto Star*, April 30, 1988.

38. Royal Society of Canada, "AIDS: A Perspective for Canadians," Ottawa, 1988.

39. "Free Condoms Suggested in Fight against AIDS, Syringes for Those at Risk," *The Globe and Mail*, April 28, 1988.

40. Terry Murray, "Epp Ends up 'Roasted' over AIDS (Non) Funding," *The Medical Post*, May 31, 1988. See also Canadian AIDS Society, "The Community-Based AIDS Movement: A Portrait of CAS," Ottawa (sent to the author by CAS in 1999). According to ACT minutes from August 1984, the idea of a national organization was raised by Dr. Brian Willoughby of Vancouver with the AIDS Committee of Toronto that month. ACT meeting minutes, Aug. 15, 1984, ACT library.

41. Michael Lynch, "Why This Die-In?" in Bernard Courte papers, accession 91-176/01, CLGA.

42. Chuck Grochmal, "Enough Talk! National AIDS Conference Shows It's Time for Confrontation," *Xtra*, May 27, 1988.

43. George Smith, "Diary of an AIDS activist," *Rites*, July/August 1988.

44. Lynch and Davis quoted in André Picard, "Demonstrators Demand Better Access to Drugs," *The Globe and Mail*, May 18, 1988.

45. Epp's quotes and STD rate changes from Canadian Press, "AIDS Programs Having Little Impact, Epp Suggests," *The Globe and Mail*, Jan. 29, 1988.

46. Kelly Toughill, "Ottawa Urged to Address AIDS Program," *The Toronto Star*, May 18, 1988.

47. Smith, "Diary of an AIDS activist."

48. Betsy Chambers, "N.S. Doctors Cool to the Suggestion of Segregating Sexually Active HIV Carriers," *The Medical Post*, Jan. 26, 1988; Dan Guinan, "Quarantine . . . Really," *Angles*, August 1987.

49. British Columbia's refusal to pay for AZT was the reason for the court action *Brown v. British Columbia* (ch. 7, n.36 here).

50. For Ontario, see Terry Murray, "Ontario Launches 2 Year $7M AIDS Ad Program," *The Medical Post*, April 5, 1988; for Alberta, see Elaine O'Farrell, "AIDS Shouldn't Be First to Get Research Money," *The Medical Post*, Feb. 8, 1988.

51. Smith, "Diary of an AIDS activist."

52. Michael Lynch to AAN! steering committee, June 14, 1988, in Greg Pavelich papers, accession 97-029/01, CLGA.

53. "IDEAS about AIDS," program 5, p.8.

54. Ibid., p.10.

eight The Charm of Politics

Interviews with Tim McCaskell, Glen Brown, Michele Brill-Edwards, Linda Hutcheon, Stefan Lynch, and Herb Spiers. Michael Lynch diaries, no. **58** (March 11, 1988–July 3, 1988), **59** (July 3, 1988–Oct. 6, 1988), **60** (Oct. 7, 1988–Feb. 23, 1989), **61** (Feb. 24, 1989–July 18, 1989).

1. Gerald Hannon, "Gay after AIDS," *Toronto Life*, November 1988.

2. Kosofsky Sedgwick also recounts this dream in "White Glasses," in her collection *Tendencies*.

3. In 1989 the Community Initiative for AIDS Research was replaced by the Community Research Initiative of Toronto (CRIT), which, in 1990, received an $80,000 award from the American Foundation for AIDS Research to conduct community-based research.

4. *Centre/Fold* I (Winter 1990) in lesbian and gay series collection, CLGA.

5. Michael Lynch to the editor, *Xtra*, March 30, 1990. After Lynch's death, his friend Ed Jackson kept the Centre alive, with a bequest from Lynch's estate, for many years. By 2000 the Centre had essentially been absorbed into the University of Toronto Sexual Diversity Studies program, which administers a Michael Lynch Grant in Queer History.

6. AAN! Press release, Sept. 15, 1988, Greg Pavelich papers, accession 97-029/01, CLGA.

7. *AIDS Action News!* 4 (Winter 1989); and "Summary Report and Recommendations: The Ontario Ministry of Health Working Conference on AIDS and HIV Infection," from Greg Pavelich papers, accession 97-029/01, CLGA.

8. George Smith to Dr. Macmillian "re: Meeting with AIDS Action Now!" undated, in Bernard Courte papers, accession 91-076/01, CLGA.

9. This definition is from an AAN! handout at the London conference.

10. In Ontario anonymous testing had been available at Hassle Free Clinic in Toronto since 1985, but the tests were illegal. It was not until 1991, after a report endorsing anonymous testing from the Ontario Information and Privacy Commission, that the provincial government provided for the expansion of anonymous testing to seven other clinics in Ontario. For a thorough discussion of the issue of placebo testing, see John Dixon, *Catastrophic Rights: Experimental Drugs and AIDS* (Vancouver: New Star Books, 1990).

11. Gina Kolata, "AIDS Researchers Seeks Wide Access to Drugs in Tests," *The New York Times*, June 26, 1989.

12. "Drug Protocol and Research Trial Working Group," in Greg Pavelich papers, accession 97-029/01, CLGA.

13. Tim McCaskell to Dr. Anita Rachlis, Nov. 27, 1988, in Greg Pavelich papers, accession 97-029/01, CLGA. For the view of the Medical Research Council, see its "Guidelines on Research Involving Human Subjects," 1987.

14. The immunotherapy approach was mentioned in a newspaper article: Alan Howard, "Many Hands Working—But None of Them Together, Einstein Would Ridicule Scattershot Approach to AIDS Research," *The Globe and Mail*, Aug. 21, 1988.

15. Michael Lynch, "Terrors of Resurrection," in George Smith papers, accession 1998-071, CLGA. The note about the "lit crit mode" and the equation were scribbled on a post-it note to George (probably Smith) on the copy of this paper at the Canadian Lesbian and Gay Archives.

16. Hutcheon was elected president of the MLA in 1999. The MLA, with 33,000 members, is the largest professional humanities and scholarly organization in the world.

17. Bruce Schentes to "Dearest Herbene, Dearest Michael, Dearest Jorgy," Jan. 30, 1989, in Michael Lynch papers, accession 91-162/10, CLGA.

18. Kelly Toughill, "Ottawa 'Doing Nothing' about AIDS, Critics Say," *The Toronto Star*, Jan. 16, 1989.

19. Ibid.

20. Health and Welfare Canada, "Pre-Market Clearance of Drug Products," Program Evaluation of the Drug Safety Quality and Efficacy Program, by R.E. Overstreet et al., Program Audit and Review Directorate, Nov. 30, 1988, revised April 19, 1989.

21. R.C.B. Graham, "Notes for Practising Physicians: How to Obtain Emergency Drugs,"*Canadian Medical Association Journal* 124 (Feb. 15, 1981).

22. A drug is used off-label when it is used to treat a condition that regulatory authorities have not approved for it. Off-label use is quite common.

23. More than a year after the program aired, Michael Hulton and the CBC were sued by the doctor who had been at the other end of the telephone line. The case was "administratively dismissed" because of lack of activity, but can be reopened.

24. Kelly Toughhill, "Experimental AIDS Drugs Released," *The Toronto Star*, Jan. 28, 1989.

25. Ontario, Ministry of Health, press release, "Aerosolized Pentamidine Centre among AIDS Initiatives totalling $7.4-million," May 29, 1989, in Greg Pavelich papers, accession 97-029/01, CLGA.

26. By February 1989 the experimental drugs made available through the EDRP for AIDS included, in addition to EL10 (DHEA), Gancyclovir, and alpha-Interferon: Ansamycine, beta-Interferon, Foscarnet, Eflornithine, Trimetrexate, Flyconazole, and Clindamnycin/Pyrimethamine. Health and Welfare Canada, Health Protection Branch, "Issues, Drugs for the Treatment of AIDS," Feb. 8 1989. See also David Adkin, "AIDS Drugs Now Available," *AIDS Action News!* 5 (Spring 1989).

27. Toughill, "Experimental AIDS Drugs Released."

28. The five-page "Dear doctor" letter finally went out on July 10, 1989, under the signature of A.J. (Bert) Liston, assistant deputy minister, Health Protection Branch.

29. A committee concerned with the rights of prisons with AIDS was formed at AAN! and then established itself as a separate organization, PASAN (Prisoners with HIV/AIDS Support Action Network).

30. Dr. Lorne Becker to Michael Lynch, April 28, 1989, in Michael Lynch papers, accession 91-162/10, CLGA.

31. Kelly Toughill, "Canada's Fight against AIDS Failing Miserably, Expert Says," *The Toronto Star*, April 16, 1989.

32. Norbert Gilmore, "Social Epidemiology of HIV Infection and AIDS in Industrialized Countries," text prepared for the World Health Organization, Working Group on Social Implications of AIDS, Vienna, Oct. 17–19, 1989.

33. Terry Murray, "Health Minister Admits: 'We Don't Have AIDS Plan Yet,'" *The Medical Post*, May 9, 1989. A month later, at the June 1989 Montreal International AIDS Conference, Health Minister Beatty told participants that Canada, lagging behind fifty countries that already had strategies, would have a national AIDS strategy by the year's end. He finally announced the strategy on June 28, 1990.

34. See Randy Shilts, "The Era of Bad Feeling," *Mother Jones*, November 1989.

35. Rex Wockner, "AIDS Activists Targeting '89 Montreal Conference," *The Bay Area Reporter* (San Francisco), Dec. 15, 1989.

36. ACT UP documents, ACT UP Archives, New York City Public Library.

37. Footage from the event is in an entertaining film about the conference by director John Greyson, *The World Is Sick*, Trinity Square Video, Toronto, 1990.

38. Kelly Toughill, "Spotlight on Canada at World AIDS Forum," *The Toronto Star*, June 3, 1989. Toughill's article begins, "When Brian Mulroney opens the world's largest AIDS conference in Montreal tomorrow, it will be the first time the Prime Minister has ever discussed the epidemic in public."

39. McCaskell quotes from Greyson, *The World Is Sick*.

40. Greig Layne, "Storming the Palace," *Angles*, July 1989.

41. In John Greyson's film *The World Is Sick*, the footage of Mulroney speaking is doctored so that, as he speaks, his nose grows, Pinocchio-style.

42. Michelle Lalonde and André Picard, "AIDS Activists Disrupt Opening of Conference," *The Globe and Mail*, June 5, 1989. For a detailed study of the activism/government relationship, see David M. Rayside and Evert A. Lindquist, "AIDS Activism and the State in Canada," *Studies in Political Economy* 39 (Autumn 1992).

43. These HIV-related opportunistic infections include CMV (cytomegalovirus), MAI (mycobacterium avium intracellulare), HIV wasting syndrome, cryptosporidiosis, and HIV encephalopathy.

44. ACT UP, "A National AIDS Treatment Research Agenda," V International Conference on AIDS, Montreal, June 1989; from a copy at ACT UP Archives, New York City Public Library.

45. Ellenberg's experience is described in Epstein, *Impure Science*, p.247.

46. AAN! "Towards a Comprehensive Federal/Provincial AIDS Policy: Policy Proposals from AIDS Action Now!" Aug. 2, 1989, in Chuck Grochmal papers, accession 97-055/01, CLGA.

47. Ibid.

48. Gary Kinsman and Brent Southim, "Draft AAN! Evaluation of AIDS Activism at the 5th International AIDS Conference," AAN! papers, accession 93-006/04, CLGA.

nine Community Strategies

Interviews with Gary Kinsman, Herb Spiers, Darien Taylor, Bill Mindell, James Kreppner, and Tony Di Pede. Michael Lynch diaries, no. **61** (Feb. 24, 1989–July 18, 1989), **62** (July 19, 1989–Nov. 18, 1989), **63** (Nov. 18, 1989–March 4, 1990), **64** (March 4, 1990–June 26, 1990), **65** (July 1, 1990–May 23, 1991).

1.   Michael Lynch, Diary, no. 61, June 25, 1989.

2.   The permanent AIDS memorial, designed by architect Patrick Fahn, was unveiled in Cawthra Park in June 1993. It appears that the 1989 memorial was remounted only once, in fall 1989, when the memorial was displayed at Toronto City Hall for AIDS Awareness Week (Oct. 16 to 20). At that point there were 484 names on the memorial, and volunteers "hosted" it, armed with a list of answers to frequently asked questions. Flyer and information sheet in Michael Lynch papers, accession 97-032/02, CLGA.

3.   George Smith, "Where Do We Go from Here?" *AIDS Action News!* Fall 1989.

4.   Footage of this blockade is in Greyson, *Pink Pimpernel*.

5.   See Paul Monette, *Borrowed Time: An AIDS Memoir* (New York: Harcourt Brace Jovanovich, 1988).

6.   Michael Lynch to Pat Lynch, Sept. 18, 1989, in Michael Lynch papers, accession 91-162/10, CLGA.

7.   Tim McCaskell, "AIDS Activism: The Development of a New Social Movement," *Canadian Dimension*, September 1989.

8.   Smith, "Diary of an AIDS Activist."

9.   Silversides, "Face It: Nice Girls Do Get AIDS." Subsequent quotes are from an interview with Taylor. After AAN! Taylor went on to co-found Voices of Positive Women, an advocacy group for women with HIV.

10. Klusacek and Morrison, *Leap in the Dark*.

11. Crimp, "Mourning and Militancy."

12. In his book *Good Intentions*, Nussbaum recounts some of the strategy and meetings between ACT UP activists and Bristol-Myers officials that led to this agreement. For Beatty's announcement, see Kelly Toughill, "New AIDS Medicine Now Available Free to Canadian Patients," *The Toronto Star*, Sept 29, 1989.

13. Nick Sheehan, "Fighting Words," *Xtra*, Dec. 8, 1989.

14. From the 1989 English Department calendar, University of Toronto archives.

15. Michael Lynch, card to "George, Ellie, Ben," Jan. 18, 1990, in Michael Lynch papers, accession 91-162/10, CLGA.

16. Michael Lynch to the editors, *The Globe and Mail*, Jan. 1, 1990 (unpublished), in Michael Lynch papers, accession 91-162/01, CLGA.

17. *AIDS Action News!* second anniversary issue, February 1990.

18. Michael Lynch, "Last Onsets: Teaching with AIDS," *Profession*, 1990, pp.32–36; reprinted in *Fuse*, Summer 1992.

19. Kelly Toughill, "AIDS Quarantine Plan Draws Protest," *The Toronto Star*, Feb. 9, 1990.

20. The reference is to a remark by poet John Berryman about fellow poet Theodore Roethke.

21. In the poem, as written in his Diary, no. 64, April 11, 1990, Lynch consistently misspelled "Alastair" as "Alistair."

22. Jim Bozyk was involved with establishing the Toronto PWA Foundation and was the subject of June Callwood's book *Jim: A Life with AIDS* (Toronto: Lester and Orpen Dennys, 1988), although in the book he was Jim St. James (he had changed his name, but he was still known in the community by his original name).

ten To Make Dying Gay

Interviews with Stefan Lynch, Ed Jackson, and James Kreppner. Michael Lynch diaries, no. **64** (March 4, 1990–June 26, 1990), **65** (July 1, 1990–May 23, 1991).

1. Lynch helped to mount a concerted letter campaign to have the HIV/AIDS lab at the University of Toronto named after microbiologist Bill Lewis. The effort was unsuccessful.

2. Clayton had at one point, apparently, publicly referred to the gay community as a "reservoir of infection." Tim McCaskell referred to this in an interview in Greyson, *Pink Pimpernel*, noting that "reservoirs are something to be drained, not treated."

3. Michael Lynch to the editors of *Outlook* magazine, Sept. 6, 1990, written on the letterhead of the Toronto Centre for Lesbian and Gay Studies, in Michael Lynch papers, accession 91-162/11, CLGA.

4. Michael Lynch, "AIDS: The First Ten Years," in the AIDS Memorial papers, accession 97-032/02, CLGA.

5. The two binders of care-team notes are now in Stefan Lynch papers, accession 2003-045, CLGA. One of his Lynch's final legacies was his care team: it, and the log book that documented activities, formed part of the basis for a care-team manual developed by the AIDS Committee of Toronto, a how-to guide for friends and family to care for someone dying at home. Rick Bébout, Yvette Perreault, and Andrew Johnson wrote the manual, *Living with Dying: Dying at Home*.

6. At some point Lynch asked Hansen to finish preparing the manuscript for publication after his death, but Hansen was not able to do this; there was not enough research gathered to complete a book.

7. Care-team notes, March 7, 1991, CLGA.

8. Care-team notes, May 9, 1991, CLGA.

9. See "White Glasses," in Kosofsky Sedgwick, *Tendencies*.

10. Care-team manual, June 6, 1990.

11. Care-team notes, June 17, 1991, CLGA.

12. Bébout, *Promiscuous Affections*, Part Five, 1987–91.

13. Care-team notes, July 4, 1991, CLGA.

14. Bébout, *Promiscuous Affections*, Part Five.

15. Lynch, "Living with Kaposi's."

16. George Smith, "Double Blind Inertia: Diary of an AIDS Activist," *Rites*, September 1988.

INDEX

Abbreviations

BL — Bill Lewis
KS — Kaposi's sarcoma
ML — Michael Lynch
PCP — pneumocystis carinii pneumonia
PWA — People with AIDS
SL — Stefan Lynch
TBP — *The Body Politic*

(federal)

AIDS Action Now! (AAN!), formation of, 131–34; first meeting, 133; beginnings, 139–41; formation announced, 145; community launch, 147–50; early demands, 150; exclusive focus, 151; social service vs. political activism at issue, 152–54; first demonstration, 156–60; strength of, 160; newsletter, 162; and Dextran Sulphate, 162–63; protest at Canadian AIDS conference (1988), 164–67; Parliament Hill demo, 168–69; successes, 177; at Conference of Clinical Trials in HIV Disease (November 1988), 179–80; general meeting and organizational matters, 178–79; Pentamidine Project, 187; prisoners' rights, 188; at international AIDS conference (Montreal, 1989), 192–95; Montreal Manifesto, 193; policy proposals, 197–98; protest about access to ddI, 206; stream of new recruits, 208; sense of urgency, 209; women in, 209; became boring for ML, 214; structural issues, 216–17; protest at Queen's Park (February 1990), 218–19

"AIDS Activism: The Development of a New Social Movement" (McCaskell article), 207–8

AIDS: After the Fear (Riordan video, 1984), 78

AIDS: A Challenge to Professionals (Riordan video, 1983), 78

"AIDS and the Arts," CBC-Radio documentary, 116; CBC-TV documentary (June 1987), 117, 174; Montreal conference panel, 196

"AIDS and the Canadian Gay Male Community" (ML and Trow document), 36, 37–38

AIDS: A Perspective for Canadians (RSC, 1988), 163

AIDS Awareness Week (1984), 77–78

AIDS Clinical Trial Group (U.S.), 197

AIDS Committee of Toronto (ACT), 22, 117, 133; origins and development of, 39–40; planning meeting, 40; early activities, 44–45; endorses name and establishes approach, 45;

first press conference (July 1983), 54–55; working with other "high-risk" groups, 54, 60–62; meeting with Red Cross, 56–57; letters patent, 61; and safe sex, 62–63; and CBC-TV's "Special Reports," 71; crises (1984), 72–73; office on Wellesley, 73–74; opposes bathhouse closures, 75; and AIDS Awareness Week (1984), 77–78, 79–80; faces financial crisis, 80–81; brochures criticized, 98–99; limitations of activities, 131; and formation of AAN! 152–54; and AAN! march, 160; treatment information exchange, 178; women's support group, 209

AIDS conferences. See Canadian Conference on AIDS; Fifth International Conference on AIDS; National Conference on AIDS; National Lesbian/Gay Health Conference; Second Annual AIDS conference; Sixth International AIDS Conference; Working Conference on AIDS and HIV

AIDS industry, 192. See also pharmaceutical companies

AIDS in the Mind of America (Altman), 105–6

AIDS Memorial (Toronto), 123, 161, 169, 171, 203, 204, 214, 228, 255n2; first memorial goes up, 172–73; ML's role in, 179; competition for design of permanent memorial, 234; argument for, 229–30

AIDS movement, 228–29. See also gay and lesbian movement

AIDS Quilt, 160–61, 173, 230,

AIDS-related complex (ARC), 56, 103, 118

AIDS service organizations (ASOS), 164

"AIDS: The First Ten Years" (ML synopsis), 228–30

AIDS Treatment and Evaluation Unit (ATEU) Program (U.S.), 155

AIDS Treatment News, 144

AIDS Vancouver, 30, 99, 164

AIDS vigils, 106, 118

Alberta, 168

Allen, Gary, 244n16

Allen, Gary Wilson, 96

Alloway, Tom, 81

alpha-interferon, 187